Dolphin Healing

Also by the same author:

Dolphin Healing

The extraordinary power
and magic of dolphins to heal and
transform our lives

HORACE DOBBS

PIATKUS

Copyright © 2000 by Horace Dobbs

Published in the UK in 2000 by
Judy Piatkus (Publishers) Limited
5 Windmill Street
London W1P 1HF
e-mail: info@piatkus.co.uk

For the latest news and information on all our titles,
visit our website at www.piatkus.co.uk

The moral right of the author has been asserted
A catalogue record for this book is available
from the British Library

ISBN 0 7499 2079 3

Page design by Daniel Mogford

Typeset by Palimpsest Book Production Limited
Polmont, Stirlingshire
Printed and bound in Great Britain by
www.biddles.co.uk

CONTENTS

Shannon's Dream

When I was born, I was normal like you
Then fate dealt a terrible hand
A mystery illness entered my brain
Now I can't talk, I can't walk, I can't stand

'Tis said that Dolphins have magical powers
And have helped other children like me
I want to go to the home of the Dolphins
I want my mind and my body set free

There are many tales spanning hundreds of years
Of the wonderful things Dolphins do
Please help me go to the home of the Dolphins
I want to be normal like you.

[Joyce Samuels]

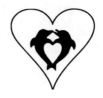

A Note from the Author

Dear Reader,

This book is presented from a personal viewpoint and its contents reflect this. So before you commit yourself to reading the entire book, I feel I should reveal how a study of dolphins and their healing powers became an all-consuming passion for me. I hope, therefore, you will at least dip into chapter 1. It will give you a taste of what's to come. It will also give you a sense of the extraordinary way events have steered me to where I am now, which, to me at least, seems more unlikely than any tale of fiction I could concoct. I feel I am still at the beginning of a great adventure.

I was born in London. I don't have a Cockney accent. I am highly qualified. As a result many people assume I come from a comfortable, perhaps middle-class background. But that, as you will discover, is not the case. I have been told by those attending my talks that I have a wry sense of humour. It sometimes comes bubbling up when I'm not expecting it, especially in adverse situations. I believe everybody should enjoy their job. If they don't they should do something different. That is why, what others refer to as my workshops, I prefer to call Dolphin Playshops. They have a serious purpose, but are spontaneous. They are places of discussion, shared experiences, warmth, vitality and, above all, laughter.

I also have a sense of mission. The realisation of this crystallised for me relatively recently. It happened in 1997 at an Alternatives meeting in St James Church, Piccadilly, in London. I had just finished giving a talk and film show on dolphins when I was approached by a member of the audience. Joyce Samuels handed me a sheet. It was a copy of an exhibit from an art gallery in London. It included a moving photograph of a little girl named Shannon and a poem (see p. ix).

I refused to read out the poem. Instead I asked Joyce to recite it herself.

I could barely speak afterwards because I was moved to tears. For me, Joyce's poem was a signpost. Immediately I heard it I knew the direction I had to take. It was to harness the love and joy of dolphins to help children.

A few days later I was contacted by Sally Galotti, an Italian artist working for Walt Disney in Milan. To me her mission seemed absolutely clear – to help children, especially those dying from AIDS in Romania. Could her talents as an artist and my knowledge of dolphin therapy be combined? I knew they could; but precisely how was hidden over the horizon.

In this book I hope to show that dolphins can provide a channel through which love can flow – both to us and from us. I want to demonstrate how dolphins have helped many people to recover from both physical and psychological illness and regain their zest and enthusiasm for life. For over two decades I have been exploring the special relationship and communication dolphins have with humans. During this time I discovered that dolphins have healing powers, and investigated this. I have also researched the possibility of artificially recreating the effects of swimming with dolphins in the wild to help those for whom this is not a possibility. *Dolphin Healing* tells a story – not just my story but those of countless others who have generously shared their experiences with me.

Perhaps Joyce's poem, or even this book, will point a way ahead for you. If this is so, I hope your journey along your personal Dolphin Road will be as joyful and rewarding as mine.

Sincerely

Horace

North Ferriby
January 2000

Chapter 1
My Story

In social-security speak, I would probably be described as coming from a background of extremely limited financial resources. When I was very young I illegally helped the milkman and delivered newspapers. Later I did a butcher's delivery round, giving most of my earnings to my mother (my father had decamped – but returned later), to supplement the family budget. I bought old bikes, painted and repaired them, then sold them. I also made wooden toys in a cupboard under the stairs that another boy, Tony Barlow, now a millionaire, sold to local shops. This was to finance my addiction – cycling. My bicycle set me free. At the age of ten I attempted to cycle on my own from Thornton Heath in South London to Brighton on an old bike with no gears. I failed. But I successfully made the 143 km round trip from home to Palace Pier and back in one day when I was 12. My reward was a brief dip in the sea wearing a pair of red woollen swimming trunks my mother had knitted for me. When I emerged from the water the dye from the wool had turned my middle regions a bright red.

Be that as it may, I was a rebellious youngster with an irreverent attitude to authority. I couldn't wait to get out of

John Ruskin Grammar School at 16. It seemed to me at the time that school work had little relevance to life in the real world. I was forbidden to associate with my best friend Ginger because we were reckoned to be a bad influence on one another – which was correct. We continued to meet of course, but secretly. That was before he was expelled – a fate I narrowly missed myself. Ginger was as mad on the air and flying as I was on the sea and swimming. He later piloted jumbo jets for an international airline. The flying highjinks of Ginger in small aircraft, before that, exceeded the exploits of the legendary Biggles. Ginger remained a firm friend throughout my life, and provided a constant reminder of the importance of following your dream.

I cycled through France shortly after I left school and paid for the ferry crossing to France from my wages (£3.25 per week) as a laboratory assistant in the Burroughs Wellcome Research Laboratories in Beckenham, Kent, supplemented with earnings from my sidelines of wedding photography and making glass animals. It was in the laboratories in Kent that I made an amazing discovery. I had always been curious about nature and how things worked. It seemed to me at the time that chemistry had all the answers – well almost. I had learnt at school how you got scum from soap in hard water and how the sugar in sugar-beet was made from carbon dioxide, water and sunlight by the process of photosynthesis. Now I discovered how you could turn a gas called ethylene into a plastic named polythene. More important than that, however, biochemistry explained how the human body functioned. It even offered a chemical mechanism for how signals were transmitted across nerve endings.

In the lab where I worked we were investigating the relationship between the pharmacological activity and the chemical structure of what were called ganglion blocking agents – the forerunners of the now widely prescribed beta blockers.

My bicycle was my sole means of transport. I cycled from home in Thornton Heath to Beckenham each morning. After work I cycled to Battersea Polytechnic in South London to attend evening classes. I got married to Wendy when I was 20. Burroughs Wellcome gave me one day a week off for study. When I was 23 I attained a BSc Honours degree in Chemistry from London University mainly from part-time study.

My next job was with the Atomic Energy Authority where I worked on a wide range of applications of radioactive isotopes. I developed an idea for a PhD thesis and found a supervisor at Oxford University. And it was in the swimming pool at Temple Cowley in Oxford that I learnt to dive as a hobby. This opened up a totally new world for me. I wrote my first book, *Camera Underwater*, which became the standard work in Britain on underwater photography for over a decade.

I had always loved swimming. As a schoolboy I often cycled to Brighton for the day, or even for an afternoon, just to go for a dip in the sea. When I became a pioneer diver I started to explore the unboundaried oceans.

It was at Oxford that my interest in dolphins really began. In my book *The Great Diving Adventure* I described how I founded The Oxford Underwater Research Group. One of our aims was to extend the limits to which humans could go under water. Through the process of evolution, dolphins had resolved a lot of the problems we were up against. They didn't get nitrogen narcosis, they didn't get the bends and they didn't suffer from hypothermia. Dolphins could travel at speed and navigate in pitch blackness. I avidly read research papers detailing investigations on how dolphins used their sonar to 'see' with sound.

However, it was not until a decade later in 1972, after getting my Ph.D and taking up the position of head of a research laboratory in Hull, that I was to get to know a wild dolphin. His name was Donald and I met him during a family holiday to the Isle of Man.

Normally dolphins swim in groups, called pods or schools, in which there is a lot of social interaction. Fishing is often a communal, co-operative activity. Much of their time is spent playing together, even in old age. When they are in the mood, dolphins will include humans in their games. If a boat is nearby they will divert and create a new game, riding the pressure wave on the bow, to the delight of everyone on board who happens to spot them. However, although it hurts our egos to think otherwise, we humans are mostly only of passing interest to dolphins. When bunched together they definitely have their own agenda. Those of us who have spent time with dolphins realise this. That is why we feel privileged when dolphins join us. Even watching dolphins at play from the shore becomes a memorable event. People often come up to me and tell of their personal magic moment. Sometimes they cannot recall the year, or even the place, but the memory of seeing the dolphins is still bright when other memories have faded.

Donald was what we now call an 'Ambassador Dolphin'. That is a dolphin who forsakes the company of his or her fellow dolphins to associate closely with humans. Being an Ambassador Dolphin makes Donald very special.

When I met Donald I was intrigued by the way he looked at me. I was instantly aware that there was something going on inside his head that I didn't know about. I knew he had a brain as big as mine. Furthermore, according to evolutionary theory, dolphins have had their big brains for 30 million years longer than humans. Admittedly a dolphin's brain is a slightly different shape, but the cerebral cortex, the highly convoluted part on the top which we associate with higher mental processes, such as appreciation of music, is more highly evolved in dolphins than it is in humans. You don't carry a big brain around in your head for 30 million years and not do anything with it, I argued. If you did, over that period of time it would have atrophied. So just what was Donald doing with that large brain of his?

Then, as if to give me a clue, one day in 1974, Donald did something totally unexpected. He picked up my 13-year-old son Ashley and gave him a ride around the harbour at Port St Mary.

Here was me, a medical researcher, with over 30 scientific papers published, watching something that could have happened 2000 years ago. A boy on a dolphin. If ever there was a sign from on high, that was it.

I desperately wanted to spend more time exploring the mind of the dolphin. But I was in a well-paid job in the pharmaceutical industry, with all that that entails. It certainly did not include gallivanting around the world probing into the psyche of dolphins.

Then, one memorable day a few weeks later, I was called in by the Medical Director who told me I was to be made redundant. Now that comes as a shock no matter what your job is. Fortunately one of the lessons I had learnt over the years was that when one door shuts, another three open. I had therefore come to look upon setbacks, especially major ones, as opportunities in disguise. Now was the time to put this philosophy to the test. I gave up the security of full-time employment, my wife volunteered to go back to work, and I set off on a trail to find out just what it was that made dolphins so special. It was the beginning of an adventure that I have never regretted for one second.

In 1978 I set up International Dolphin Watch (IDW). It is still flourishing as a non-profit organisation dedicated to the care and understanding of dolphins – especially their relationship with humans.

One of the people I observed to be profoundly affected by Donald the dolphin was Geoff Bold, a mechanic at Penlee Lifeboat Station in Cornwall. Geoff was close to a nervous breakdown and the dolphin lifted his blues. His full story is told in my book *Follow a Wild Dolphin*. I also made a film about Donald for Yorkshire Television, *Ride a Wild Dolphin*, which was directed by Barry Cockcroft (see page 184).

At the end of the film I commented that dolphins have an aura, or give out an emanation, that makes people joyful. At that time I couldn't explain it, but I was convinced dolphins could change a person's state of mind. Just as I was starting to formulate ideas on how to investigate this, Donald disappeared without trace. At the time records of lone dolphins that interact with humans in the sea were extremely rare. I could find no accounts between AD109 and 1955. Thus, statistically, the chance of finding more than one of these special dolphins in my lifetime appeared microscopic.

Even so I set off on a quest to find another friendly dolphin and explore the undersea world. It was a mission that was not without its more exciting moments. These included being attacked by bandits whilst sailing on an Arab dhow in the Persian Gulf, and becoming shipwrecked in the Philippines.

My search took me far and wide. I had some brief encounters with a dolphin named Dobbie in the Red Sea in 1980 and recounted these experiences in *Save the Dolphins*. Sadly Dobbie was killed shortly afterwards by a shot from a rifle. Then in 1982 I made contact with a dolphin called Percy in Cornwall. Percy's interactions with a woman called Tricia Kirkman were to affect me profoundly.

Tricia, who was shortly to become a grandmother, had a history of emotional problems. She couldn't swim and had never even been in a swimming pool. Yet she plucked up courage to put on a wetsuit and go into the sea half a mile off the coast of Cornwall to swim with a dolphin. Shortly before she had her first encounter, the dolphin, who weighed over 200 kilograms, jumped back and forth over my head as I bobbed in the water.

This display of acrobatics was awesome for me. Not surprisingly for Tricia it was not conducive to self-confidence. When she slid slowly into the water she was absolutely terrified. What happened next was one of those moments of dolphin magic that has stayed with me ever since.

Tricia floated nervously in the sea, buoyed up by her wetsuit. Percy hovered quietly under her and allowed Tricia to place her hands on his back. Then, very gently and slowly, he towed her in a circle around the boat. When we hauled her back onboard Tricia sat on the rubber wall of the inflatable boat with her legs dangling in the water. As she did so the dolphin reared his head out of the sea and rested it momentarily on Tricia's lap. She bent down and kissed the glistening domed head, whereupon the dolphin withdrew and went quietly about his business elsewhere.

It was obviously an intensely moving experience for Tricia. Afterwards, when I asked her about her feelings, tears poured down Tricia's face. She said she could give the dolphin nothing, yet she felt that Percy gave her love. Unconditional love. I later discovered that Tricia was immensely sensitive and had had a very turbulent emotional life including being raped. For the first time in her life she had been loved and nothing was expected in return.

When the film I helped to make about Percy was shown on television, the BBC was inundated with mail. Many of the letters were from viewers who suffered from depression. They reported that the programme, *Eye of a Dolphin*, had lifted their spirits.

The following year Tricia and I went to Wales to make a film for HTV about a solitary young dolphin, Simo, off Solva in Pembrokeshire. Whilst there I was approached by the daughter of a man suffering from chronic depression. She asked if I would take her father to see the dolphin. She explained how her dad, Bill Bowell, had become depressed following a heart attack and the wrongful accusation that he had stolen from the restaurant he managed. So we took Bill out to see Simo the dolphin (for more, see my book *Dance to a Dolphin's Song*).

When Bill got into the water something uncanny happened to him. His melancholia vanished. When Tricia commented that Bill had 'blossomed like a sunflower' the seeds for a new International Dolphin Watch research project, *Operation Sunflower*, were sown. Its aim was to see if dolphins could help those suffering from clinical depression.

Seeing what happened to Bill, I was convinced that dolphins also had something to offer humanity. Just what it was I couldn't say. But I knew, deep down, that I had stumbled, apparently by accident, on a mysterious yet powerful force that could transform human lives – especially those of the chronically depressed.

Chapter 2
Dolphin Dreamtime

In 1986 a solitary, friendly dolphin, Fungie, was frolicking with those who cared to join him in the sea off the fishing port of Dingle in County Kerry in Ireland. I had decided to use this location for the launch of Operation Sunflower, to test my theory that dolphins could help the clinically depressed. Bill Bowell was one of the people involved in the investigation. The others I chose were Jemima Biggs, whose depression presented as anorexia nervosa, and Neal Jackson who suffered from paranoia.

The television film I made for TVS about my experiments was called *The Dolphin's Touch* (see page 183). It showed how Fungie responded to the three depressives when they swam with him. More importantly, it showed how *they* responded to their encounters with the dolphin. I fully accepted that my study in Dingle did not fulfil the criteria for a proper clinical trial. (After receiving my PhD in 1968 and being elected a Fellow of the Royal Society of Medicine, a rare honour for a non-medic, I became involved in clinical trials and became acutely aware of the enormous amount of evidence in the form of scientific data that had to be gathered before any claims for efficacy could be established.) Nonetheless I was absolutely convinced that I was on the right lines.

With the benefit of over ten years' hindsight, I can now see that each of the patients involved in that first experiment in Operation Sunflower made an important contribution to my understanding of the manner in which dolphins can help those with psychological illnesses.

Firstly there was Neal Jackson, a young man in his early twenties who had a life-long history of paranoia. When I introduced him to Fungie I told Neal the dolphin would do him no harm. But Neal didn't trust me, or anyone else. In his mind everyone and everything was conspiring against him. Consequently when Fungie appeared out of the blue-green underwater haze, Neal thought the dolphin was a shark. He was so scared that he bit right through the plastic spiggots in the mouthpiece of his snorkel tube, and swallowed them. Even when I tried to reassure him, Neal was still very suspicious and nervous. But he had made his first step to overcoming his paranoia. When we returned the following year Neal's self-confidence had grown and he had lost his fear of Fungie completely. He jumped into the sea and zoomed around the dolphin as playfully as a seal.

I can now see that letting go of fear is one of the ways in which dolphins can help humans, and not just those with clinical paranoia. Whether we openly acknowledge it and recognise it or not, fear, in one form or another, is present in all of us – without exception.

When we first took Jemima Biggs to Ireland her body was severely deprived of nutrition. A young woman also in her early twenties, her anorexia had been exacerbated by the death of her grandmother. To conserve her resources, nature stopped Jemima having her menstrual periods. Jemima also found it difficult to have very close personal relationships. Yet two years after swimming with the dolphin, although she still had problems eating, Jemima got married and later produced two healthy children.

How did this come about?

We all have days when we are down. It is quite natural. What Fungie showed Jemima was that there could be highs in life, as well as lows. Again, this is something we should remember, and can all take benefit from, when we feel our personal skies growing dark.

Thirdly, there was Bill Bowell, the chronic depressive. For 12 years he lived in what he called 'the black hole of depression' from which there was absolutely no escape. When Bill swam first with the dolphin Simo, then with Fungie, he saw some light. Since then he has described publicly the heart-rending story of how, aided by his wife Edna who he now describes as his 'land dolphin', he climbed out of the dark hole to resume a normal life. He takes no medication or other treatment. The opposite, in fact. He is now dispensing treatments to others in the form of encouragement. Those he talks to often respond to him more than to doctors because he knows what they are suffering. His clinical card might well say 'spontaneous remission'. I would not disagree with this. But I would add a rider – 'with the aid of a dolphin'.

The lesson I have slowly learnt from Bill, and from other cases like his, is that we all have an ability to heal ourselves. But we need help to do it. That help can be a dolphin in a physical form, as it was with my three volunteers. Alternatively, and sometimes just as effectively, the dolphin encounter can be purely imaginary. I discovered this later when I took a journey into Dolphin Dreamtime.

The success of my study in Dingle posed a major problem. An estimated one person in ten in the Western world was expected to need some form of psychiatric help during his or her lifetime. Thus in Britain alone there were, potentially, five million people who might possibly want to swim with a dolphin. Clearly taking even a tiny fraction of these people out into the sea to swim with dolphins was utterly impossible.

I needed a dolphin pill. But as no pharmacological interactions were taking place, what possible form could my non-chemical pill take?

The Australian Aborigines had the answer to my quest for a dolphin pill, Dolphin Dreamtime. I discovered that with the aid of music, they could take a listener into a mental state akin to that of an encounter with a dolphin.

At first I found the whole concept of the Dreamtime extremely difficult to comprehend. So many aspects of Aborigine culture were completely alien to my Western, achievement-motivated way of thinking. Animals, vegetables and minerals were not separated into different categories. The Aborigines were not competitive. They had no concept of possessions. Their continent was criss-crossed with songlines. You could not own land, but you could be the custodian of the song that brought the land into existence and 'marked' its boundaries. Even the Aborigines' concept of time was completely different. In the Dreamtime, the past, the present and the future were fused into each moment. To the Aborigines every animal had a spirit that could be more important than its physical reality.

I was intrigued when I heard about the Dolphin Dreamtime cassette in which the listener is guided into the sea to swim with the dolphins, via a journey through a cave full of beautiful crystals. It is written by the healer Taranath Andre, and the narration is overlaid with music by Glenda Lum whose totem is a dolphin. Instead of a didgeridoo Glenda uses a synthesiser that is more familiar to Western ears, supplemented with real whale and dolphin sounds.

When I first listened to the tape, in the dark whilst floating in a pool, I had an extraordinary, out-of-body experience. I had the sensation of water flowing across my body as I swooped into the depths. I was a dolphin. I knew what it was like to be a dolphin. The heavy feeling that had prompted me to go for a swim evaporated in a flash. When I later asked those attending one of my playshops at the College of Psychic Studies in London to listen to the tape, they also had out-of-body experiences. What was even more extraordinary was that each person had a different experience. This convinced me that somehow or other Dolphin Dreamtime captured the essence of an encounter with a dolphin. I decided, therefore, to see how a wider audience would be affected.

Via International Dolphin Watch I made the Dolphin Dreamtime cassette available to members on a random basis. Each cassette was supplied with a confidential questionnaire which was returned to me. Analysis of the first responses at the Applied Psychology Unit of the Medical Research Council in Cambridge in 1990 was sufficiently encouraging for me to extend the trial. A 12-page statistical analysis conducted by Richard Pearl in the Department of Psychology at Swansea University of the 173 responses received up to 1994 indicated that over 70 per cent of those listening to the Dolphin Dreamtime benefited from the experience.

Investigative journalists, including Pat Pryor (BBC Radio 4) and Anne Page (*The Guardian*), evaluated Dolphin Dreamtime. They confirmed its efficacy in the treatment of stress-related illnesses. So I had my dolphin pill – an audio pill in the form of a cassette.

In 1997 a support worker for the learning disabled sent me a eulogistic account of the benefits the Dolphin Dreamtime was bestowing upon her, her colleagues, and her clients. She concluded the letter with the comment 'I am living proof that dolphins help to heal wounded spirits'.

Dolphin Dreamtime, which is distributed as a tape and CD by International Dolphin Watch, is now established as a useful tool in psychiatric wards. In addition to helping those diagnosed as clinical depressives, Dolphin Dreamtime is finding ever-widening applications. These range from post-operative trauma and pre-examination relaxation, to tension release in prisons. A doctor uses it to help himself deal with his own disability – myalgic encephalomyelitis (ME). So far there have been no contra-indications.

Responses to Dolphin Dreamtime continue to arrive, often from unexpected sources. In 1999 I received a letter from Australia, beautifully handwritten by a former Research Associate of the Smithsonian Institute in Washington, in which she thanked me for a tape I had sent her in 1992 and described how following the death of her dog she 'became severely depressed again, and in this period the tape reached into the depths of my sadness, as a ray of light'.

In 1999 I also received several reports, based upon long-term observations, on the sometimes profound benefits of Dolphin Dreamtime in childbirth. These prompted me to initiate structured studies, starting in 2000, which will provide scientific data to support the accrued anecdotal evidence for the value of both real and simulated dolphin encounters in childbirth – from pre-conception to post parturition.

Jeanette Pickering, a mother of four, who had derived immense personal benefit from Dolphin Dreamtime, agreed to undertake a study of the value of Dolphin Dreamtime in antenatal clinics. For Jeanette dolphins are symbols of spirituality. Roma Todt, a midwife, also agreed to take part. She and her husband Volker will take pregnant women to swim with dolphins in the sea from their dolphin-watching boat based in The Canary Islands.

Chapter 3
Arion and the Dolphin

Once I had embarked on my dolphin trail of discovery, I could never envisage being in full-time employment again. The value of freedom was one of the first lessons I learnt. Just as the bicycle set me free from the straitjacket of an impoverished childhood in a soulless suburb of London, and the aqualung released me from being stuck on the surface of the sea like a cork, so the dolphins liberated me from the constraints of political politeness and scientific correctness which are a pre-condition of employment by large companies. The total freedom I had to explore new scientific concepts, and more importantly to express openly my views on such issues as whale hunting, which I was forbidden to do by my employers because of the effect this might have on the sale of their products in Japan, only became apparent to me later.

From my very earliest memories, until the present day, life has been a continual and often surprising learning process for me. No more so than when I stumbled, entirely by accident, on the fact that dolphins could help people suffering from depression. Discovering that the healing spirit of the dolphin could be captured with Dolphin Dreamtime was another revelation. What I find exciting about dolphin healing now is that I do not know where it will lead in say 100 years' time.

I am encouraged to think this far ahead because in 1999 aspirin celebrated its 100th birthday. It's origins are as real, yet tantalising, as figures half hidden in a mist.

Magical properties have long been attributed to the willow tree. As early as 400BC Hippocrates, the father of medicine, recommended willow bark infusions to ease labour pains. Gypsies made a drink from willow bark for easing rheumatism, influenza and headaches. Then along came organic chemists to whose ranks I once belonged. They discovered that the primary active ingredient in willow bark is salicylic acid which in its pure form is very useful for relieving pain, but the side effects are unpleasant. These are considerably reduced in a derivative, acetyl salicylic acid, which has the common name of aspirin.

And so, in March 1899, Bayer launched Aspirine®, or aspirin. It has since become the most widely used pharmaceutical in the world. An estimated 60 billion doses are taken every year. Eleven thousand tons are consumed annually in the US and Britain alone. Consumption continues to rise as its use for protection against heart disease becomes more widespread.

When looking for new remedies, the first step many researchers take is to review folk law. In the case of dolphins it is abundant. Dolphins have always had a special place in human hearts. Dolphins are surrounded by mythology. In Ancient Greece to kill a dolphin was punishable by death. The stories of them helping humans are legion. Clearly ancient people had a deep respect for these marine mammals. Did they know, perhaps subconsciously, that dolphins had healing powers?

This thought was certainly in my mind when I was approached in 1992 by Rebecca Meitlis of English National Opera (ENO) to see if I would be interested in co-operating with the Baylis Programme on a community opera based on the classical story of Arion who was saved by a dolphin. I knew the story well. I couldn't resist.

Rebecca endeared herself to me immediately when she argued that she couldn't really commission an opera about Arion if those directly involved had never had an experience that came remotely close to swimming with a dolphin in the open sea. I offered an immediate remedy to this situation. The entire team, with myself included of course, should adjourn for several months to a remote tropical paradise. Hawaii, for example, where we could pass the days languishing in the company of schools of dolphins. Rebecca pointed out that sadly the budget did not stretch that far. Indeed it didn't stretch very far at all.

When I told her how a dolphin off the coast of Ireland had transformed the lives of Bill, Jemima and Neal, she agreed that Fungie should be able to wield his magic equally well upon a team of talented artists about to embark upon the creation of a new opera. A short time later a small group assembled in Dingle.

As we scrambled aboard a fishing boat laden with tourists, I wondered if the dolphin would appear. If he did would Fungie, who I hadn't seen for nearly a year, recognise me? What kind of reception would I get if I got into the water with him? Questions buzzed through my head as we headed out of Dingle harbour.

Suddenly, just beyond the harbour wall, a face reared up alongside the boat. The sun glistened momentarily on the shiny, silvery dome of the dolphin's head. There was a loud 'phtt'. The dolphin submerged. The next moment the sea erupted. Like a launched missile, Fungie soared into the air. Higher and higher he rose. His flight path curled. For a microsecond of real time, but etched forever in my memory, the dolphin hung, suspended like a pewter statue against the sky, his streamlined body curved into an archway above our heads. Then he plummeted down, thwacking into the sea with an almighty splash.

For less than a heartbeat the garrulous crowd on board were stunned into silence. Then they erupted with noise. Some of them shook their clothes to flick off the water that had cascaded into the boat when the dolphin splashed down alongside. Others, their faces streaming with water, screamed with delight and surprise. Like supporters of a football team when a winning goal is scored in the final seconds of a match, they roared their ecstatic approval. Children jumped up and down shrieking with delight.

Everyone onboard had come to meet a wild dolphin in the open sea. They had been warned that as he was totally free there was a chance they would not see him at all. Now, out of the blue, Fungie had come to see them. That one display of acrobatics more than satisfied their greatest expectations. Even if they never saw Fungie again, their trip to Dingle had been worthwhile.

Fungie had come up trumps again. The group from ENO were spellbound. We were on our way to creating a wonderful new opera. The story of Arion and the Dolphin would be told yet again. And in the retelling of the classical myth, I hoped I could take another step towards uncovering the ancient secrets of the dolphin's healing powers.

Chapter 4
Project Vision

My very first visit to see the dolphin in Dingle had been back in 1985, shortly after he had begun to build up a strong association with humans and a year before I was to take Bill, Jemima and Neal to meet him. As more and more people swam with the solitary dolphin, so the stronger his bond with humans became. At first he was dubbed Dorad – the Gaelic word for dolphin, given to him by English visitors. This left-brained derivation of a name was far too twee and logical for the Irish, who eventually settled for Funghie, and then Fungie, which is easier to spell. I asked several of the local fishermen why the dolphin was called Fungie, which to me sounded like a kind of fungus – hardly an appropriate name for a lovely dolphin. It was obvious that none of them knew. It just happened.

But one of the things the Irish are good at is spinning yarns, especially in pubs, of which Dingle has many. During my trip with the ENO, I heard a beauty.

'What kind of name is Fungie for a dolphin?' I asked a fisherman who was sharing the bar with me.

'Well, it was like this sur,' he replied in his wonderful

southern Irish accent. 'We get a lot of forin boats coming into this beautiful harbour of ours. One day we had a boat come in from Italy, we did. Your man, that's the dolphin sur,' he added in explanation, seeing that I was foreign, 'went out to escort the boat in. And doesn't he do that for all the boats coming into our harbour?' He paused for dramatic effect. 'Well, one of the crew spots the dolphin and gets very excited, like he would. Sure, at the time aren't they passing the headland. An Italian fisherman looks up and sees lots of mushrooms growing on top of the cliffs. "Fungie," he cries. That's the Italian word for mushroom sur. When the rest of the crew hear him shouting "Fungie" they think it's the name of the dolphin, they do. That night in the pub aren't they telling everyone about Fungie. The people in the pub wouldn't be after telling the Italians they'd got your man's name wrong would they? Especially as they were so excited at seeing the dolphin they're buying everyone drinks.'

I nodded in agreement.

The fisherman drained his glass and placed it carefully and deliberately on the bar. He wiped the froth from his lips with the back of his hand, and, like the Ancient Mariner, fixed me again with his gaze. He did so with the earnest sincerity of a man about to give me a hot tip for the next runner in the Derby. 'So you see sur, that's how the dolphin got the name of Fungie.'

I couldn't argue with him. He paused and slid his empty froth-rimmed glass a few inches across the bar, a subtle gesture that did not go unnoticed.

'You mark my words, sur,' my new found friend continued, 'one day this dolphin of ours will be as famous as the dolphin in that opera of yours.'

I asked him what he would have to drink.

'A pint of Guinness would do very nicely sur,' he said.

Fungie's fame spread far and wide. One of those who furthered this process was a dear friend of mine, the poet, playwright and actor Heathcote Williams. Heathcote was very sensitive. He had black days himself and understood the problems of the three depressives when we were together filming *The Dolphin's Touch* in 1986. Heathcote stayed on in Dingle, taking photographs and writing. One outcome of his endeavours was his epic illustrated poem *Falling for a Dolphin*.

> As you move through a world without boxes, or walls, or
>   doors, or roads,
> With no one ever between you and the sky,
> Leaping through three dimensions towards whatever takes
>   your fancy,
> You would be different.
> And close to,
> Drawn into the dolphin's force-field,
> Smitten by the shamanistic glimmer
> In an eye that distils a life-long exposure
> To another, rarer state of things,
> You too are alchemically touched.

Another person to hear of the antics of a friendly dolphin in Dingle was Cheryl Hutchins. She had become blind following the onset of diabetes. Her husband Mike was her carer and their son, Stephen, who had cerebral palsy, was confined to a wheelchair. Cheryl and I corresponded via cassette tape recordings. She had a gentle, mellifluous voice that conveyed no indication of the problems she faced every day. Cheryl had a powerful desire and a strong reason to swim with Fungie. These had originated some years earlier following visits the family had made to Brighton and Windsor Dolphinariums.

People often ask me about dolphins in captivity. I tell them that for me the situation is akin to that of human slavery. When slavery was rife we did not know, or care to accept, that all humans, regardless of their origins, have a right to freedom. The situation changed when William Wilberforce and others campaigned for the freedom of slaves because they felt the practice was immoral. Now that principle, of a right to freedom for all men, is accepted almost universally.

In my view a similar situation now exists with regard to dolphins in captivity. Many people, especially those who have worked closely with dolphins, feel that freedom is a right for the mammals who have been dubbed 'man's cousins in the seas'.

Knowing my strong views on this issue it was with some slight misgivings that Cheryl Hutchins told me about her encounter with a dolphin in Brighton Dolphinarium. It was an experience that was to change her life. She felt sure a dolphin named Silver singled her out when she sat on the side of the pool after the show. Cheryl told me she and Mike both sensed that the dolphin knew she was blind. Cheryl used touch instead of sight to explore what was around her. Silver encouraged Cheryl to stroke her all over, including her flippers and blowhole. A similar situation occurred at Windsor, where Winnie the killer whale even allowed Cheryl to put her hand inside her cavernous mouth, and rub her tongue. As a result of these magical experiences, Cheryl and Mike decided to investigate non-verbal and non-visual communication between humans and dolphins. They collected remarkable stories indicating that dolphins could tell when a human was disabled, or when a woman was pregnant, and would then seek out such people specially.

I explained to Cheryl that it would suit my stance admirably if I could say that dolphins in captivity did not have a powerful effect on the human psyche. But I knew from innumerable stories that, even when held prisoners, dolphins still radiated a feeling of joy that sensitive people picked up immediately. It was irrepressible. Perhaps that in itself was a lesson for us humans. Resentment, bitterness, or a burning desire for revenge appeared not to exist in a dolphin's nature.

Cheryl and I had long, and for me, stimulating conversations on many aspects surrounding human/dolphin relationships. We debated the unconditional love that I had seen shown to Tricia Kirkman by Percy in Cornwall, and the startling effect Fungie had had on Neal, Jemima and Bill. We came to the conclusion that the anecdotal evidence was much more than coincidental. The dolphins seemed to know who needed help. One way of accounting for this was to assume that dolphins were telepathic.

During one of our many discussions Cheryl made a statement which seemed to be at variance with her personality. 'Horace, one of the first things we must all learn, is to love ourselves.'

At first I found this comment unacceptable.

'I don't agree with that. Surely the opposite applies,' I said. 'We should not focus on ourselves or become egocentric. That makes us selfish and inconsiderate to others.'

'No, that's not what I mean at all,' explained Cheryl patiently. 'We should love ourselves for what we are. Not be dissatisfied with our lot. Be happy with our bodies – no matter what shape they are. Of course we can and should seek to improve ourselves. But at the end of the day *be happy being you.*'

In hindsight I think that this is one of the most valuable pieces of advice I have ever been given.

I have thought about what she said many times since. I've decided it is one of the characteristics of dolphins that appeals most to me about them. I feel they are happy to be dolphins and do what dolphins do best, which is to have fun, even in difficult circumstances. Don't ask me how I know this. I just feel it inside. An essence of self-fulfilling joy radiates from them like light. I am sure it contributes to their healing power.

However, Cheryl, Mike and I were not in Dingle to investigate Fungie's powers of healing. Together we had set up *Project Vision* as part of the International Dolphin Watch research programme. It's aim was to look at non-verbal communication and see if Cheryl could establish some kind of telepathic bond with Fungie. Wetsuits were purchased and Cheryl learnt to snorkel in the local swimming pool.

Cheryl and Mike were in Ireland in June 1992, the same time as the group from the ENO. A film crew from Germany arrived too. Getting the two snorkel divers and the camera crew geared up took some time. Fungie liked action and didn't hang about if nothing much was happening. By the time Cheryl and Mike were ready to go into the sea, he had disappeared. We tried revving the engine, which usually attracted his attention. But Fungie declined to come back. Mike and Cheryl decided to go in anyway in the hope that the dolphin would return. They had practised a code of hand squeezing to signal to one another.

When Mike and Cheryl slid into the water I had no doubt that Fungie was aware of their presence. He would sometimes appear from the other side of the bay within seconds of somebody paddling into the sea. But would he come back to Cheryl and Mike?

With the loss of sight many people develop a more acute sense of hearing. What would Cheryl hear if or when he came near? Would she hear more than the squeaks I had heard Fungie make? I watched them snorkel down and disappear from view. We would have to wait until Cheryl returned to find out what she was experiencing.

Chapter 5
Seeing with Sound

When I first took up diving I read a book by the co-inventor of the aqualung, Jacques Yves Cousteau. It was called *The Silent World*. I quickly discovered, however, that the underwater world was far from silent when I listened in to the sea with an underwater microphone called a hydrophone. The sea sounded noisier than a city street. I was absolutely amazed at the variety and clarity of the sounds. With the use of appropriate sound filters it was possible to select and amplify selected signals. This is something the brain can also do. For example we use selective hearing, mentally cutting out the background babble, whilst listening to someone in a noisy, crowded room.

A hydrophone depends upon a membrane that vibrates in air, like the human eardrum, to produce a signal. However, when I read about the complexity of dolphin hearing I realised that all a hydrophone could do was give me a tiny insight into the dolphin's world of sound. In addition to the sounds I could pick up with a hydrophone, dolphins could hear sounds outside my hearing range. They generated and listened to the echoes of high-frequency sounds that I couldn't hear. These they used for echo location and echo inspection – i.e. *to see with sound*.

At first the best I could do when trying to appreciate how dolphins perceived their sounds was to think in terms of the ultrasonic scans I had seen of babies in the womb. Slowly it dawned on me that the blurred black and white images were inadequate and possibly completely misleading.

As I watched Cheryl and Mike disappear into the waters of Dingle Bay I knew full well that Fungie was as aware of what was going on around him in his underwater world as we humans were in ours. But whereas we humans use vision as the main source of information, dolphins depend mainly on sound. The reason for this is the obvious one of limited visibility underwater, which at times can be virtually zero.

The most widely accepted explanation for the presence of dolphins on our planet is that they are the descendants of quadrupeds that once roamed the land. The development of an ability to see with sound, ie echo locate, was one of the most remarkable evolutionary adaptations made by dolphins when they made the transition from land to water.

When submarines were introduced into warfare, seeing with sound underwater became more than a scientific novelty. It was a military priority. The acronyms ASDIC (Allied Submarine Detection Investigation Committee) and SONAR (Sound Navigation And Ranging) came into common use. Research was intensified when nuclear submarines, armed with guided missiles, became major tactical weapons in the Cold War between the US and USSR. In the US in the 1950s and 1960s military money was available in the form of research grants. Not surprisingly scientists focused their attention on dolphins who had built-in detection systems far more advanced than any man-made devices. A plethora of scientific papers appeared which demonstrated beyond doubt the remarkable echo location and echo inspection capabilities of the dolphins. These included being able to find fish and then tell the difference between one fish and another in complete darkness.

Around this time I was working at the Atomic Energy Research Establishment (AERE) at Harwell, in Berkshire. The research work on dolphins fascinated me for many reasons. Among them was my interest in the detection and measurement of all forms of radiation – both ionising and non-ionising. As far as I was concerned visible light and audible sound were two very different types of radiation.

Light falls into the category of what is termed non–ionising, electromagnetic radiation. It is generated by oscillating electrical and magnetic fields. These electromagnetic fields, like gravity, exist throughout the universe. Visible light is just a tiny part of an extensive band of such radiations which can be defined by their frequency and wavelength. The band extends beyond the blue end of the spectrum to include ultraviolet and microwaves. The red end of the spectrum stretches to longer wavelengths that include the radio waves. This vast spread of electromagnetic waves, all of which have different characteristics, have one thing in common. They travel at the same speed. The speed of light in fact.

The speed of light in empty space is about 300,000,000 metres per second. We talk about the inconceivable distances between our planet and the stars in terms of light years. Such light radiation, which can traverse the universe without absorption and may take years to reach us, is stopped in a nanosecond by a sheet of black paper. At the instant of impact it is transformed into another form of vibrational energy – heat.

Sound radiations, on the other hand, have completely different properties. They travel at different speeds, governed by the equation: speed = frequency x wavelength. The speed of sound is microscopic compared with light. It varies with density, elasticity and temperature. In air the speed of audible sound is a little less than 340 metres a second. This explains why in stormy weather we see lightning, which travels at the speed of light, before we hear the thunder, which of course travels at the speed of sound.

The relatively slow speed of sound enables humans to tell the direction from which sound is coming. This is achieved by the brain being able to identify the tiny difference in the time it takes for a sound to reach the ears, which, being separated, are slightly different distances away from the source. Underwater these differences in the time of arrival of the signal are too small for the brain to differentiate, because sound travels four times faster in water than in air. Thus humans cannot tell where sound is coming from underwater. Dolphins obviously can however.

Sound also travels much further and much more clearly through metal and water. I found this out by chance myself one day whilst taking a bath. I put one ear under the water when someone was tapping the pipes in another part of the house. The sound was very loud and crystal clear when my ear was submerged. Yet when I lifted my head clear of the water I could barely hear it. This mini discovery enabled me to understand more readily the concept that dolphins, and especially large whales, can use sound to communicate over vast distances underwater.

The human ear can only detect sounds in a limited frequency range, usually from about 100 up to 15,000 cycles per second. Sounds below this range, called infrasounds, and those above it, called ultrasounds, cannot be heard by us. But some of them can by other animals. The high-frequency dog whistle and bat sonar are examples.

As I watched and waited for Mike and Cheryl to return I pondered briefly, once again, on the mechanism by which dolphins can hear. I have an eardrum, the timpanic membrane, which vibrates in air. These vibrations are transmitted via tiny bones to the cochlea, which in turn generates signals which are passed on to my brain via the auditory nerve. In order for the eardrum to vibrate there has to be an open passage between the source of the sound and the timpanic membrane. If I want to block out sound, I wear earplugs. However earplugs do not eliminate sounds completely. Other parts of my body can pick them up and pass them on to the cochlea, bone conduction being the most effective.

Dolphins do not have an outer ear for gathering sound, like most mammals. Indeed, the outside opening, the external auditory meatus as it is called, is barely visible. It can sometimes be seen as a tiny indentation behind the eyes. There is no clear air passage between this external ear and the modified eardrum. Instead, sound signals are transmitted via body tissue from the outer ear to the inner ear. A surrounding barrier of oil helps to insulate this pathway. However, this is not the sole route for the transmission of sound signals. Because of their direct contact with the surrounding water, sound vibrations pass right through a dolphin. Thus, in addition to hearing sounds via their ears, dolphins perceive them through their bodies. In other words, dolphins are bathed continuously in sound, and their entire bodies are sound receivers.

The bones in the flippers of a dolphin correspond to those of the human hand which is sensitive to loud sound-pressure waves. This raises the interesting possibility that a dolphin's flippers are sound antennae as well as hydrofoils.

People who are blind often have an enhanced sense of hearing to compensate for the loss of their sight. It was therefore with mounting anticipation that I waited to find out from Cheryl what she experienced when she heard Fungie. The film crew were excited too. They knew that Cheryl had had an encounter with Fungie because they had seen the dolphin suddenly surface near her when she was underwater. Fungie then dived in such a deliberate way that he was obviously going down to inspect her.

'Well, what happened?' I asked when Cheryl and Mike were both safely back in the boat.

'I saw him briefly,' said Mike.

'I know you did,' said Cheryl. 'I felt you squeeze my hand.'

'Did you hear him?' I asked.

'Oh yes,' said Cheryl. 'I heard him. But I saw him too.'

'What do you mean? Saw him? You're blind!'

'I didn't see his shape. I saw colours just before Mike squeezed my hand. There were lots of them. They were unearthly.'

'That means you were aware of the dolphin before Mike saw him,' I replied excitedly.

What Cheryl said made sense. Fungie would have been using his sonar as he approached the two divers. Mike couldn't see Fungie, but Cheryl could detect the arrival of the dolphin with her sense of sound. What was absolutely fascinating, however, was that she interpreted this sound as colour. When I quizzed Cheryl about them she said they were unlike anything she could remember from the time when she could see.

This was an exciting observation. It meant that sound signals could be interpreted as visual images in the human brain. Subsequent research by psychotherapist Dr Olivia de Bergerac and her partner William MacDougal in Australia revealed that dolphin interactions caused shifts in brain-wave patterns. These bands, or ranges of electrical brain emissions, are represented by Greek letters which do not follow a logical sequence. They are assigned as follows: delta, below 3.5 cycles per second (cps); theta, 4.5–7.5 cps; alpha, 8–13 cps; and beta, above 13 cps.

The higher frequencies are active during normal daily activities and are associated with action, concentation and problem solving. Too much beta activity is indicative of stress, anxiety and burn out. The lowest frequencies are produced during deep sleep and coma.

The theta waves have been linked to the so-called twilight state, between waking and sleeping. These theta frequencies have been correlated with mental activities such as reverie, sudden insight, free association, creative ideas, problem solving etc.

One of the responses reported after the use of theta brain-wave neurofeedback therapy has been spontaneous imagery or hypnagogic imagery. Thus the colour images perceived by Cheryl may now be explained by the high-frequency sounds emitted by Fungie interacting indirectly or directly with her brain, and causing a shift in brain-wave emissions.

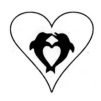

Chapter 6
Liquid Bliss

The proposal for Mike and Cheryl's plans to investigate the way blind people might be able to detect and possibly interpret the sounds made by dolphins was first announced in the January 1992 issue of the International Dolphin Watch magazine, *Dolphin*. The same issue of the magazine carried a letter from Wendy Huntington to the editor, Melanie Parker. It revealed how Wendy and her husband Tony had decided to blow their savings on a trip to the clear blue, warm waters of the Bahamas after reading an article about a psychotherapist called Rebecca Fitzgerald and her experiences with dolphins in an earlier issue of *Dolphin*. Rebecca organised trips for people who wanted to swim with dolphins.

Dear Melanie and friends

I have been unwell for seven to eight years, possibly ME, and suffered from bouts of depression since my early twenties. Last year I sought the help of people in the fields of various natural therapies and the culmination was the dolphin trip this year.

We met some wonderful American friends on the dive boat; we were the only Brits – how brave we were!?

Since my return, I feel lighter and have more energy. I have been able to resume my early morning swims three times a week and I am in love with the universe. It is a joy to be alive.

Up to 1991, Operation Sunflower had been focused on the role dolphins might play in the relief of clinical depression. I had heard that Dr Betsey Smith, a psychologist from Florida, had observed that swimming with dolphins produced improvements in children with autism. I did not know at the time that this was an area of dolphin therapy in which I would become increasingly involved later. As Operation Sunflower unfolded, anecdotal evidence started to filter through to me that the healing effect of dolphins might have other applications. Wendy Huntington was a case in point. ME (myalgic encephalomyelitis) is a inflammation of the brain and nervous system that causes pain, muscle weakness and a general feeling of wretchedness that comes and goes. The etiology of ME is uncertain but it is thought to be viral in origin. It usually comes under the category of psychosomatic illnesses – that is medical conditions with physical or somatic symptoms that arise from mental problems which cannot be precisely defined. Whatever the cause, the outcome is very distressing. It often strikes people who lead very active lives and stops them from engaging in sport and other activities that incur physical and mental exertion. So to hear that dolphins had helped Wendy Huntington completely regain her previous zest for life was exciting news indeed. It also raised lots of questions. How did it work? How long would the improvement last? I put these two questions to Rebecca Fitzgerald and she gave me her personal written account of Wendy's story.

During the summer of 1991, I got a call from a woman in England named Wendy Huntington. Wendy had been suffering from suspected ME for eight years and had heard that swimming with dolphins might have some curative affect on her condition. Hoping for a cure, she rang me up to see if there were any slots available for her and her husband Tony to join us. Luckily, we had room on an August trip and they booked passage right away. As they began preparations for their trip we had several phone conversations about Wendy's physical condition and whether or not she would be strong enough to go. The trip from London to the Bahamas involved several airline transfers and two overnight stays in a hotel; she was worried that she hadn't the stamina. I encouraged her to come.

When I met Wendy in person she was feeling pretty tired from the journey. We all had dinner together at Port Lucaya in Grand Bahama the night before our morning boat departure and she explained to the group that the virus had left her with symptoms of fatigue, nausea, muscle cramps, insomnia and some depression. She had heard Dr Horace Dobbs give a lecture on the possibilities of dolphin healing and, since none of her medications were working, decided to give it a try.

Around 8.00am the next morning, our group of 16 met in the hotel lobby and walked over to the boat which was to be our home for the next five days, out of the sight of land.

About five hours later we were in our bathing suits, out at sea and cruising around in the general dolphin area. We eventually dropped anchor and people either went for a swim or remained on board talking and enjoying the sun. By late afternoon we were visited by part of the dolphin pod who were swimming nearby and wanted to say hello.

As usual, we spotted their dorsal fins cutting through the light blue sea as they swam straight for the boat. Some of us got in the water immediately to let them know we were there and ready for a swim.

It took Wendy a few minutes to get her gear on and enter the water from the back of the boat. It meant donning an underwater mask, snorkel and fins, then going over the back of the boat to climb down seven or eight stairs of a ladder to get to the dive platform resting just above the water's surface. She managed to enter the warm Bahama waters and join the others swimming with the dolphins.

Wendy was a good swimmer so she had no trouble keeping up. Within minutes she was surrounded by wild dolphins; a group of glistening grey bodies, dark spots and beautiful soft eyes. She wasn't alone, we were all in the water by now, 16 people in a large, loose group, accompanied by dozens of dolphins swimming above, below and beside us. It was an experience of liquid bliss; of synchronistic swimming and blended energies of human and dolphin.

As usual, the encounter came to a close as the light was leaving. The sun sets around 8.00pm in the summer and as we swam back to the boat we watched our beautiful ocean friends jump and leap and somersault away. It was the end of a perfect day as we all sat down to supper to share our experiences.

Each day brought new adventures. Some days the dolphins came early, at 6.00am. Other times they wouldn't show up until dusk as we waited impatiently, keeping constant vigil fore and aft, port and starboard. As always I reminded everybody not to make the dolphin encounters the only focus of their trip. There is much to harvest from these expeditions and exchanges with the dolphins are only a part of it.

Wendy, however, had but one thought. Her desire to find relief from ill health was foremost in her mind and she was tremendously hopeful that the dolphins would assist her in this process. I was cautious in my explanation of how and why dolphins have an impact on us and their healing influence. I didn't want to give rise to false hopes but I had seen several people experience physical and emotional healing after swimming with these dolphins and felt it was important to make that information available.

Several days into the trip we had a marvellous encounter with a couple of dozen wild dolphins. It was late in the afternoon and as we were sitting on the back deck chatting and watching the water surface for signs of dorsal fins, we spotted the group heading towards us from the west. They were leaping out of the water as they splashed their way to the boat. We had plenty of time to get our gear on so everyone was already in the water by the time they reached us. Our hearts were beating fast as we felt the wave of approaching dolphin energy. The sea was filled with sound; clicks and whistles and high-pitched squeals were ringing in our ears as sleek, grey bodies zoomed past us, under us and made a circle around our group. They swam among us, giving each person plenty of time to fully experience their presence. It was thrilling, it was exciting, it was beautiful and it was timeless. So timeless that I didn't notice the sun going down, eventually sinking below the horizon. The sky was turning its usual shade of lavender/blue/grey and the water surface began to reflect the light instead of being clear. It was time to head back.

The boat crew saw that the current had carried us away from the ship and considered getting an inflatable boat out to bring in the weaker swimmers. Instead the captain powered the boat round in a big arc, arriving in the area of the swimmers, who gradually climbed aboard, apart from Wendy. She was now well away from the boat, but swimming steadily in our direction. Wendy's husband Tony, having been in the water earlier, was standing on deck next to the ship's captain. The captain asked if Wendy would be OK or whether they should fetch her in. Tony replied, 'She'll be fine, just let

her swim in, she's obviously enjoying the experience.'
We all watched Wendy steadily pull herself through the
sea, one stroke at a time. It wasn't an easy swim; the wind
picks up a bit in the evening and the water surface was
choppy. Also, the current was flowing against her so she
had to keep moving forward. No rests were possible.
Stroke by stroke, arms constantly pulling her through the
water, Wendy brought herself to the boat.

When she arrived at the dive platform Wendy was
absolutely glowing. She pulled herself up onto the
platform then climbed up the ladder to Tony and me
waiting on the deck.

If her countenance was any measure of healing, then
indeed, Wendy was well again.

Without saying anything more, she went below to
shower and dress for dinner. Tony and I just looked at
each other without knowing what to say. At dinner that
night, she explained her reasons for not wanting to be
picked up out of the water. Although it appeared that
the dolphins had left the area, they were simply out of
our eyesight and were broadcasting sound into the
water. Unbeknownst to us, Wendy's body was
responding. She felt the sonar penetrate her skin and
pulse through her entire body as it began to bring her
into what she described as a 'balanced and exhilarated
state'.

Wendy was in the water being pulsed by the
dolphins' sonar for about 45 minutes. From the boat I
couldn't hear the sounds being emitted by the dolphins
and was unaware of what Wendy was experiencing. I've
been in the water when it's filled with dolphin sonar
and the feeling is that of being a musical instrument; an
instrument that's being perfectly played. The vibrations
move through our tissue and bone and palpate us at our
deepest levels.

I can honestly report that Wendy was different after this
experience with the dolphins. She was, in fact, radiant.

Her energy was bright, her spirit was renewed and she was infectiously happy for the last two days of the trip. The woman who ended this Dolphinswim was not the same woman who started it.

Having got a record of the event from Rebecca, my scientific background kicked in. I asked Wendy to give me her personal account of what happened. This is what she wrote:

After a very long swim back to the boat, I climbed out of the ocean tired yet energised. I later closed my eyes. I saw a long corridor with doors on either side in colours of the rainbow. They were all ajar, and one by one they opened wide and disappeared. I was left with a warm, open space where I could move and dance freely without anyone or anything holding me down, or back.

Whilst in the water I was totally unaware that the rest of the group had left, because the sounds in the water at first baffled me. It sounded like seaweed popping and squeaking, as it does off the shores of the British Isles. However, there wasn't any seaweed, so I just kept my head down in the water and absorbed the wonder of the moment. I just *was*. Anything else happening wasn't touching me. It was only when I intuitively lifted my head, that I realised I was quite a distance from the boat and everybody else was back on board! There was no fear, only a renewed strength, freedom and peace. So I gave a wave to the boat, put my head down and swam back!

This experience with the dolphins led me to understand that I was able to absorb from them something that enabled me to heal a part of myself. A 'feeling' rather than an intellectualisation! It appears to be an exchange of information that occurs when an individual is ready and open to receive. You feel, enjoy and are 'in the moment'.

I came home to England and was accepted as a

student of homoeopathy. My health was very good until
the beginning of the fourth and final year, when I had
two viral infections. These were followed by another
bout of ME or chronic fatigue syndrome, which
continued for four years.

I felt the dolphins had shown me a healing direction.
I just didn't get it quite right, so I had to take another
turning.

The turning Wendy took was to qualify as a reiki master. She
also learnt the Metamorphic Technique and embarked on the
first Oceantherapy course in Europe devised by Sergi Aymo,
during which she was instructed on the multifarious ancient
and modern, mystical and scientific healing benefits conferred
by the sea itself and the life forms that inhabit it, especially
dolphins.

Wendy pointed out to me that 'a healing' was not
necessarily 'a cure', yet she felt very strongly that 'the dolphin
spirit', as she called it, was still directing and guiding her life.
On one point she was absolutely certain. Wendy felt really fine
again and was looking towards the future with excitement and
enthusiasm.

Chapter 7
Drenched with Happiness

Wendy was so thrilled with the outcome of her swim with the dolphins that in 1992 she invited Rebecca Fitzgerald to come to England and give a presentation in Chesterfield Public Library in Derbyshire. I was invited to attend. In the slide show she presented that evening, Rebecca held me spellbound with her tales of spotted dolphins.

Rebecca's story began in 1984 with a strange experience when she was in the final year of a master's degree in psychotherapy at a college in Santa Fé, New Mexico. It happened in the middle of the night. Rebecca was dreaming about dolphins covered with speckles. Suddenly she woke up. Her eyes were open. Rebecca was fully conscious, but no longer in her bedroom. She was in the sea. Wide awake, she was experiencing the same scene she had just been dreaming about.

'The water was turquoise blue, not very deep. I was floating on the surface while two spotted dolphins jumped hoops around me. My mood was joyous. I lay happily on the surface while they whistled and cavorted around me,' she told us.

Rebecca was relaxed yet had a heightened sense of awareness. She knew she was in her bed in the dark. Yet at the same time she was submerged in warm water in the company of two dolphins.

Gradually the scene faded and she felt herself only in bed. After several minutes sitting up in the dark she went back to sleep. When Rebecca awoke the next morning she felt somehow connected with dolphins, and was filled with a great sense of enthusiasm.

A similar thing happened the next night. This time, however, there were many more dolphins. The sea was alive with their sounds. What interested Rebecca most was that this was not a new experience. It was an old one. It was as if she was somehow connected with her ancient past. In repeated awake dreams Rebecca retained a close connection with the dolphins for the next ten nights. They did not confine their visits into her conscious mind to the hours of darkness. The dolphins swam around her during the day.

'I hasten to mention that I was not on drugs of any kind,' she pointed out forcefully. 'But I was very curious about what was going on. I went to the public library. Like most Americans the only dolphin I was familiar with was Flipper, a grey bottlenose dolphin with no distinguishing marks. He certainly wasn't covered with speckles. I thought the spotted dolphins were a figment of my imagination.'

Much to her surprise, Rebecca discovered that there were lots of different species of dolphin, not just the Flipper variety. Then, there they were. A photograph showed a group of small spotted dolphins, *Stenella attenuata*, swimming in clear turquoise water. This unnerved Rebecca. She felt delight and confusion at the same time.

'I wanted to shout out loud that the images in my dreams were real dolphins. But I had no idea where the images originated. I left the library in a daze.'

The dolphins then started to come into Rebecca's conscious mind in what she described as 'lucid dreaming' just before she went to sleep. What was more, they now communicated with her in words.

'As I moved from wakefulness to sleep they began instructing me. As I hung in the water they would swim into a shape, perhaps an octagon, with myself at one corner. They told me to "feel" the shape. It was as if they were giving me a lesson in space and time. During this lucid dream state I was a mathematical genius. I grasped all the concepts and understood the shapes in a holistic way. It was as if each shape had a sound and colour. It was a great game and I played it with unbounded enthusiasm. It was fascinating how each construct had an impact on my physical self. The feeling of a triangle differed greatly from that of a square. I had definite preferences.

'One night, after a particularly exhaustive session, I heard a voice say "Write this down. We're giving you specific information and you are forgetting the precision of it when you wake up." I kept a pen and notebook beside the bed to help with my post-graduate studies. So I dutifully promised to record my instructions and promptly fell back to sleep.'

Rebecca kept her word. When she woke up she wrote down what she was told, which were often complex mathematical formulae. The dolphins offered Rebecca the idea that they had known one another for a very long time, and that their relationship was far beyond the physical. Rebecca was very comfortable with this integration of spiritual with the physical.

'I was happy and at home with these dolphins. In fact I was experiencing a unique combination of ecstatic bliss and peaceful fulfilment. The only other time I'd felt such a deep sense of connection was when my daughter, Maria, was born. Although I was pregnant for only nine months, I'd waited a whole lifetime for her to show up. I knew it the moment I saw her. The dolphins had the same kind of impact. Their appearance seemed sudden and unbidden. Yet I felt a huge portion of my deepest self finally slip into place. What impressed me most at this time was that I awoke each morning drenched in happiness. My energy level increased. I felt more alert. Although I didn't know it at the time, I was beginning an entirely new chapter in my life.'

Rebecca was a month away from graduation. The dolphins were a total distraction. She told herself very firmly that it had to stop. And, like switching off a switch, it did. And Rebecca went on with her life in the usual way.

After she graduated, Rebecca had a successful career in psychotherapy. She practised what she had been trained to do. It worked to a degree, but not as well as she hoped. She knew she could do better. Something was always lurking in the back of her mind. It disconcerted her. She believed, like the famous Swiss psychologist Carl Jung, that most of the people who came to her for help were sick because they were unaware of, or cut off from, spiritual experiences and understanding.

Then, quite suddenly, four years after she had graduated the dolphins came back. She began having flashbacks, during meditations, to the most positive aspects of her childhood, like giggling in the double bed with her sister on Saturday mornings when there was no school. These were joyful aspects of her past she had completely forgotten about. After one such meditation a pod of dolphins was swimming around the ceiling of her bedroom.

'What are you doing here?' demanded Rebecca.

What happened next was to change Rebecca's life.

'I began to understand that the processes I went through in my own therapy and therapy training had focused on pain, and had concentrated on behaviours learnt through suffering. There was a relentless scrutiny of dysfunctional experiences, and repeated reporting of distress and hurt. The dolphins seemed to be saying that they wanted me to re-experience the positive aspects of my childhood, not the painful ones. They stimulated my memories of sweet, tender moments. I began rethinking my childhood.

'The most memorable thing which happened that night was that I heard the dolphins say, "You choose your memories. *Choose again!*" I was left sitting in bed with those words echoing in my head. They were offering joy, and I was offering sadness. I was astonished at how much of my youth I had completely forgotten.'

Later I found out that Rebecca's early life had been unusual to say the least. Her grandfather was a pure Cherokee and would often wander off for weeks or months at a time. Her father was a homosexual and desperately tried to hide his sexuality even when Rebecca was an adult and her parents were divorced. Rebecca's father was rich. Her mother scraped a living singing. In the school holidays she lived in her father's luxury house. The rest of the year was spent in relative poverty with her mother.

'I've had a large percentage of joy in my life but I had convinced myself that my father's alcoholism and mother's depression overshadowed everything and that I was hopelessly involved in sadness and misery. Even more astonishing is that I didn't know I believed that. It had just gradually become a subtle part of my thinking and world view. That night my life changed. It took a while for the insight to sink in and become an integrated part of my consciousness, but the actual shift happened quickly.'

At the time this happened, Rebecca had started to take small groups to swim with captive dolphins in the Florida Keys. Then she heard about a pod of wild, free dolphins in the Bahamas. She booked a passage on a research vessel to meet them. Rebecca became progressively more excited as she recounted the next part of her story.

'After a storm that lasted all night, I awakened to the same energy I'd felt in 1983 when the dolphins first approached me during sleep. The other passengers were asleep, recovering from a rough night of tossing and turning and vomiting. I'd slept in my bathing suit and when I felt the dolphin energy coursing through my body/mind, I quickly rose and climbed the ladder to the deck.

'Only one man was there, the staff naturalist, who offered to pour me a cup of coffee. It wasn't yet 6.00am. I told him the dolphins were coming, that I could feel it, and he chuckled, rolling his eyes and shaking his head in amusement. He bent over to grab the coffee thermos on the floor, and as he did so, I could see, over his bent back, at least 12 dorsal fins cutting through the blue water, heading straight for our boat.

'I yelped like a kid and ran over to the side, pointing at the dolphins streaking toward us. Since he was dressed in blue jeans and a heavy sweater, the naturalist couldn't get in the water right away. The other passengers were below, sound asleep. After getting his permission to enter alone, I jumped over the side with my mask and fins already on. No sooner did I plunge under the surface than I was surrounded with dolphins and the full effect of their incredible sound. Just like the dreams, I was engulfed in a wave of dolphin energy and cadence. They swam in fast circles around, below and above me. I cavorted with them for over half an hour.

'I was in a state of bliss. I lost all sense of time or limitation. I swam better, stronger, faster and longer than I ever had in my life. There was no weakness or sense of being tired. I'd never felt more myself than I did for those 30 minutes. If there was ever a sense of "coming home", this was it. Years of discomfort, sadness, confusion and disorientation fell away. The great sense of wakefulness that I experienced during the dreams in 1983 became my physical reality. There, in the turquoise waters of the Bahamas, surrounded by wild spotted dolphins, *I was reborn.*'

After her first, half-hour, ecstatic encounter Rebecca calmed down. She had barely finished focusing her thoughts when the dolphins, who were floating quietly beside her, exploded into action again.

'They jumped and spiralled and somersaulted with glee. The water turned to white bubbles, and I couldn't see a thing, but I could hear the high-pitched whistles and clicks. The water was alive and filled with activity. I thought my heart would burst. I swam like a woman possessed.

'I dived down and then kicked as hard as I could to propel myself up and out of the water. I curled into a ball as I dived back down and did innumerable somersaults under the water. I squealed with delight and grabbed handfuls of sand at the bottom. I was out of my head! The rejoicing was uncontrollable and it continued until I was completely out of breath. I'd exhausted myself beyond my physical limits. It was then that I noticed how far from the boat I'd gone. The vessel looked small. I realised I had a long swim back.'

The dolphins escorted Rebecca as she dog-paddled back to the boat. She was exhausted but not nervous. The crew had been watching her. They had an inflatable on hand and could come and pick her up immediately if she needed help.

As she made her way back Rebecca's head was filled with messages from the dolphins, to return and bring people with her. 'We will honour you with our presence' were the last words she heard as she pulled herself up the ladder to the dive platform on the stern. It was a request she couldn't refuse. It was time to change.

Rebecca abandoned the methods of psychotherapy she had been taught. For Rebecca helping her patients exorcise their problems by getting them to relive past painful events was not the way she wanted to proceed. She would pioneer an alternative method involving joy, not anguish.

Everyone has emotional problems that they have to deal with sometime in their lives. Henceforth she would help them to find the plateau of joy on which the dolphins existed. To do that she would take groups to swim with the spotted dolphins that roamed across the Bahamian sandbanks. Wendy Huntington and her husband Tony were just two who bore witness to the fact that she had made the right decision.

As I listened to Rebecca's spellbinding stories, I speculated once again on the unexplored territory that my scientific background didn't deny existed, but which hitherto I had viewed from afar with hesitancy and scepticism. Could Rebecca and her spotted dolphins lead me, and those I was trying to help, into another reality? Up on to another plane of living where love reigned supreme? It seemed wildly idealistic. But past experience had taught me that, where dolphins are concerned, dreams really can come true. Future events were to prove it yet again, when Rebecca introduced me to the spotted dolphins in the Bahamas.

Rebecca's indication that dolphins had access to special knowledge that we have since lost, intrigued me. What were the formulae that they had given Rebecca? Did they contain clues about how ancient civilisations, like the Egyptians, 5000 years ago, could cut and move stones weighing 20 tons with an accuracy that would be difficult to match today with all our machines and technology? And what about Atlantis, the ancient civilisation believed to be lost beneath the sea. Did it exist? Could the dolphins lead me there? As it turned out Rebecca was to be instrumental in setting me on the road to explore that particular question in 1997 off the island of Bimini in the Bahamas (see chapter 20).

Of course, I did not know that as I sat in the Public Library in Chesterfield in 1992. When Rebecca had finished her talk there was one question, like a fuelled-up rocket about to be launched into space, that I was burning to ask. 'Can I see the books in which you wrote the information given to you by the dolphins in your lucid dreams?'

'No, Horace, you can't,' she replied with a disarming smile. 'You won't believe this, but I've lost them!'

Chapter 8
Looking to the East

In truth, when I met Rebecca in 1992, I had already made a major step along the road towards an explanation, if not a full understanding, of dolphin healing. And it would not have been possible if I had stuck rigidly to the objective and scientific approach to medicine prevalent in the West.

Like most of the big events in my life it happened with little forethought on my part. At times I feel as if I am a pawn in a jolly game being played by 'The Man Upstairs'. Not that I am opposed to this situation. I just do what feels right, regardless of what arguments might be waged against it. For some reason, which is completely beyond me, every year since first meeting Donald the dolphin and adopting this travel-in-trust approach, life has become progressively richer, more exciting and more rewarding. So when I was asked if I would like to attend a conference in a monastery to be held in April 1991 in the Italian town of Cortona, all expenses paid, and give a talk and a playshop, I didn't have to think about it for long. With wine and food on offer *ad libitum*, and the thought of Italy in spring, I felt it would be churlish to decline the invitation. So I accepted on behalf of my wife and myself.

~~Dolphin~~ *Dolphin Healing*

The offer came about as the result of the generosity of a rich Swiss industrialist. He felt that new graduates and doctorates coming out of Swiss universities were too narrow in their outlook. He wanted to broaden their horizons. In order to achieve this he financed a week-long gathering once a year at which they could meet and mingle with renowned experts of different disciplines, from around the world. There was a strong leaning towards the arts. When I saw the eminence and accomplishments of the other speakers, I had a sneaking suspicion that someone must have dropped out, and I was a fill-gap. All the presentations had to be given in English on a single theme. This particular year the theme was metamorphosis. I felt that the metamorphosis of a caterpillar into a butterfly had been adequately covered by the authors of numerous biology textbooks. I therefore opted to recount, with the aid of film, the changes that had been wrought upon me, and others, during my personal metamorphosis from atomic scientist to dolphin devotee.

I included a clip of the film I had made about Donald in my one-hour presentation. I was on good form. When I concluded, a small solitary figure stood up in the audience. Tears were streaming down her face.

'I am Shizuko Ouwehand,' she said. 'This afternoon I am supposed to give a workshop on calligraphy, but I cannot do it now because it is at the same time as Horace's workshop on dolphins. I have been much moved by Horace. He has touched my dolphin button. I *must* go to his workshop. May I therefore, with respect, ask all of those who were coming to my workshop to go to Horace's dolphin workshop, sorry playshop, instead?'

Shizuko did indeed come to my playshop and brought her calligraphers with her. It was the beginning of a friendship that I cherish beyond measure. If ever there was a dolphin in a human body it is Shizuko. She is one of the most generous, joyous natural healers it has been my privilege to meet and through her my research into dolphin healing has been greatly enhanced and advanced.

When I 'touched her dolphin button', as Shizuko expressed it, I made her fully conscious, for the first time, of a deeply rooted connection with dolphins that had been hiding inside her since childhood. Once her 'inner dolphin' surfaced, Shizuko couldn't suppress it. It jumped out of her body.

Shizuko's feeling of attachment to dolphins was so strong she considered it to be part of her genetic make-up, so I asked her if she had heard of Elaine Morgan. She hadn't.

Elaine Morgan is the author of a book called *The Aquatic Ape* in which a powerful case is made for a period of aquatic adaption, followed by a return to the land, as part of our evolutionary history. I told Shizuko that I had discussed this concept many years ago with the man who first propounded it, the late Professor Alister Hardy.

'Does that mean dolphins and humans really are connected?' asked Shizuko.

'It could do, if the aquatic theory of evolution is correct.'

I went on to explain that it was a controversial topic and that the existence of this kind of connection could explain why some people have such a strong affinity with dolphins.

'It's irrational really,' I continued. 'Some say we are attracted to dolphins because they smile. They don't smile. Dolphins have a fixed jaw line. They live in what to humans is an alien environment, the sea. Dolphins are shark shaped. We should be terrified of them. But we are not. We instinctively love dolphins. And that love goes both ways.'

'So could there actually be some kind of genetic link?' asked Shizuko.

She also wanted to know if there was any other evidence for the apparently irrational bond between humans and dolphins. I told her about another book, *Mind the Waters: A Book to Celebrate the Consciousness of Whales and Dolphins*, published in 1974, that had opened many thought doors for me. It contained two chapters on dolphin brains. One of them was by Myron Jacobs, the one-time Director of the Cetacean Brain Laboratory of the New York Aquarium. The other was by Peter Morgan who, with Myron Jacobs, mapped out the dolphin brain. Jacobs' contribution was entitled _The Whale Brain: An Anatomical Basis of Intelligence._ There was also a fascinating chapter by Sterling Burnell on the evolution of cetacean intelligence. An idea that had been around for some time was that the growth of a foetus in the womb retraced the path of evolution for that species. In the chapter by Burnell there was a collection of drawings of the foetuses of a white-sided dolphin that showed a startling resemblance to that of a growing human embryo. When I later photocopied the chapter and sent it to Shizuko, I underlined the following:

> Dolphins have a higher neocortical–limbic ratio than even healthy, intelligent humans, and captive dolphins and orcas have often shown humour, empathy and self-control that few of us could match under comparable circumstances. As Fictelius and Sjolander have suggested, we humans depend on highly adaptive cultures in which most of the mental capacity lies outside the individual and in the traditional knowledge of the culture. As regards our brain and our capacities as individual conscious beings, we may actually be inferior to some other kinds of large-brained animals.

Alongside this paragraph was a quote in bold type. **You see, what I found after 12 years of work with dolphins is that the limits are not in them, the limits are in us.**

This statement was from arguably the father of dolphinology – neuroanatomist John Lilly. His books, such as _The Mind of the Dolphin_ played a large part in the change in our thinking about dolphins which, up until the 1960s, were widely regarded simply as animal clowns in aquatic circuses.

I suggested to Shizuko that the concepts expressed by Burnell and Lilly indicated that dolphins have perhaps overtaken us in some respects on the road of evolution, and we might have some catching up to do.

Shizuko, in turn, opened a thought door for me. When I

told her that I could find no explanation compatible with my knowledge of Western medicine to explain dolphin healing, Shizuko politely asked if I had cast my eyes to the East. 'No,' I responded. When I said I had never heard of ki (pronounced kee), Shizuko said 'Ki is the same as qi'.

'The concept of qi is the cornerstone of traditional Chinese medicine,' she added.

Traditional Chinese medicine, Shizuko explained, has a totally different philosophy to that of Western medicine. In old China you paid a doctor to keep you healthy. If he failed you stopped paying him. So it was in his interest to keep his patients in full health all of the time. In other words they practised preventative medicine.

Shizuko went on to explain other differences. 'In the West you give your medical students a corpse. He or she then dissects out the various organs and builds up a picture of the human body based upon these observations. They learn pharmacology, chemistry, etc and use this collective knowledge, often with synthetic drugs, to treat their patients.'

I nodded in agreement.

'In the East we have a different approach. We learn more about natural healing processes. We ask "what is the difference between a living body and a dead body?" The answer is qi, which is the essence of life. We are imbued with it when we are born. It then flows freely through our bodies throughout our lifetime. If that energy flow gets disturbed, illness results. So the student doctor learns how to get the energy flowing freely again using special natural preparations and acupuncture.'

I had heard about acupuncture but the rest was new to me.

Shizuko continued. 'In the West when a doctor first sees a patient he or she usually uses a sphygmomanometer to measure blood pressure and a stethoscope to listen to the heart and lungs. They are symbols of his office if you like. In the East the first diagnosis is usually done by looking at the tongue. Doctors must learn to identify medical problems from hundreds of different states of the tongue. Having made a provisional diagnosis the next thing the Chinese doctor probably does is to attempt to get the energy flowing smoothly again. This he does using acupuncture needles, for instance. They are the symbols of office for a Chinese doctor.'

I realised, of course, that this was a very simplified version of the fundamental differences between Eastern and Western medicine. This became clearer to me when I later read Ted Kaptchuk's book *Chinese Medicine* which looks at all aspects of Chinese medical theory through the eyes of a sympathetic Westerner. As Shizuko had pointed out to me, Eastern medicine sees health and disease quite differently from Western medicine. In the East the treatment of illnesses is more philosophical. In the East, illness is a disharmony of the whole body. An essential element of Eastern medicine is therefore that the part cannot be considered in isolation from the whole. For example, if you have a migraine you cannot just think of it as a problem associated with the head. It must be looked at in relation to the entire body.

Another book which greatly helped me understand what Shizuko was trying to tell me was *Encounters with Qi: Exploring Chinese Medicine* by David Eisenberg with Thomas Lee Wright. In it Eisenberg, a graduate of the Harvard Medical School, describes his extraordinary experiences at the School of Traditional Chinese Medicine in Beijing.

Listening to Shizuko and reading the books did not radically change my opinions on Western medicine, much of which I thought was good. In the field of orthopaedics, for example, especially when coupled with high-tech diagnostic procedures such as computerised X-ray scanning, the West excelled. We were superb at replacing worn hip joints and mending broken bones. However, when it came to the kinds of medical problems that could possibly benefit from dolphin healing, often referred to as psychosomatic illnesses, it seemed to me that the Chinese approach provided an alternative that merited serious consideration.

Shizuko suggested I meet her ki master, Dr Nakagawa, to see ki therapy in action. I was all for it.

Between stays in Japan Dr Masato Nakagawa was constantly on the move, touring the world and generously giving healing sessions in places he felt they were especially needed, such as Chernobyl in Russia where people were suffering radiation sickness. Dr Nakagawa also regularly presided over week-long courses at his special centre for ki healing in Shimoda on Japan's Izu peninsula. Here his patients gathered for collective treatment, and he trained others in his healing techniques.

Dr Nakagawa had started life as a watchmaker and founded a school of watchmakers for handicapped people. When electronic watches started to appear he realised that his future prospects were limited. He had powers of healing which he apparently inherited from his father. He started to practise ki healing which had been almost completely discontinued as his country slavishly followed Western methods of medical treatment.

Dr Nakagawa coupled his engineering and design skills with his healing methods and developed and improved machines that generated ki. This added greatly to his success. His followers could now be treated with impressive looking ki machines with dials and moving needles, as well as getting treatment directly from the master himself. Money flowed in. Dr Nakagawa was offering alternative treatments to the Western methods that totally dominated health management in Japan. Not surprisingly, he was regarded as a threat especially when he openly stated that Western methods were often inappropriate, and usually much more expensive than his. The pharmaceutical industry demanded that he should substantiate his claim, validate the efficacy of ki, and prove that his machines generated it. Dr Nakagawa couldn't do this. Furthermore he stated that he had personally to endow his Hi Genki machines with his consciousness in order for them to generate ki. This, said his detractors not surprisingly, amounted to witchcraft.

Unable to prove his claims, Dr Nakagawa was charged and sentenced to a term in jail where he set to work healing his fellow inmates and wardens. Eventually the prison governors and their families were attending his healing sessions. When he was eventually released his following was greater than ever.

During his six-week stay in prison, Dr Nakagawa discovered he could transmit ki energy through the walls to prisoners in other cells. This led him to the realisation of distance healing, whereby he could transmit ki to any part of the planet.

Within a few months of meeting Shizuko, I was invited by Dr Nakagawa, via Shizuko, to attend and give a talk at his 100th Natural Healing Seminar in Tokyo. The seminar took place in a room packed with about 300 of Nakagawa's students and patients who had come to learn and be treated with ki energy. They were of different ages with a wide range of medical conditions. Before I spoke Dr Nakagawa performed a healing. It was the first time I had seen collective healing, and it was a culture shock, to say the least. With his fingers outstretched and pointed towards his audience, he waved his arms in a kind of fanning movement to the accompaniment of music. The effect on his audience was instant. They all shut their eyes. Some rocked from side to side. Others waved their arms in the air like Eastern dancers. It was altogether bizarre. I was the only Westerner in a room filled with people who had left their bodies and gone into a state of ecstasy. I waited.

As I did so a young woman rose from her seat and, with undulating and gyrating movements of her body, made her way to where I was sitting. At first she waved her hands back and forth across the dolphin image on my sweatshirt. Then she pressed her thumb on to a small pile of dolphin books I had stacked on the table in front of me. She clutched one of them between her fingers and thumb and remained doing so until Nakagawa finished his treatment and swept his hand quickly over the top of her head. The movement brought her out of her trance. When she opened her eyes, her fingers were still locked on the book. She could not release them. Shizuko said she could keep the book as a gift. The young woman bowed to Shizuko, and to me, then walked back to her seat.

Seeing my bemused expression, Shizuko explained to me that the lady in question was highly psychic and that what she was picking up was the ki force of the dolphins – not so much from me, nor from the dolphin emblazoned across my chest, but from the words and pictures in my books.

Back in my hotel room later that night, I pondered whether dolphin images really could carry their own healing power. And was it the case, as Dr Nakagawa believed, that dolphins and whales naturally emitted ki and played a vital role in keeping mother earth healthy? I had plenty to think about.

Chapter 9
Shimoda and the Quest for Ki

I was intrigued by the concept of the life force, or universal energy, that Shizuko called ki. Its pervasiveness sent a tingle through me.

'If ki is the answer to dolphin healing, then we've cracked it,' I told Shizuko triumphantly. 'If I can give a logical explanation for ki, with scientific back-up, dolphin healing will become more acceptable. We must set up a research programme, observe what happens to patients, and measure ki. The measurement of ki is vital.'

Shizuko's reply took me aback. 'Measure ki. Why do you need to measure ki? Everybody knows it works. No need to measure it.'

'That may be so in Japan,' I told her. 'But it isn't so here. We Brits want proof. Real proof. We have to be able to measure something for it to be accepted as real. It's built into our mental programming. It's no good just saying it's a hot day. We want proof it's a hot day. We are distrustful. The person telling us may want to sell us a refrigerator. Television programmes constantly tell us the world is full of charlatans. We want to know precisely what the temperature is, in figures. Then, we are convinced,' I said cynically.

It was a poor example to quote, but it was the first one I could think of. It was superfluous anyway. Shizuko, who was married to a Dutch university professor, was totally aware of the differences between Eastern and Western culture.

She then gave me a brief lesson on aspects of philosophy which centred around the concept that *the more precisely something can be defined, the less valid it becomes.*

This was one of those ideas that as a scientist I first dismissed as absolute poppycock. It seemed to me, at the time, to run contrary to everything I had been taught – to the very foundation of science itself.

Once Shizuko had placed the thought in my mind, however, I mulled it over, time and time again. I realised that I was in danger of being dogmatic. There was a lot of quiet wisdom in the East. Life experiences were teaching me that science didn't have all the answers. I was not the only one, however, who was keen to find positive proof of the existence of ki. Stephen Rose, who produced documentary films for BBC TV, was interested in alternative medicine and was sympathetic to dolphin healing. The kind of investigative programmes he made required masses of research beforehand and concrete evidence of efficacy.

Stephen and I knew from experience that he would need to provide much more proof than anecdotal evidence of ki energy and its connection with dolphin healing before the BBC would seriously consider making a programme that would fit into one of the well-established para-scientific slots in their schedules. The kind of programme Stephen Rose had in mind required input from many different sources. We were all keen to see such a programme made. But how could we provide the scientific proof necessary for the project to get the go-ahead?

Stephen obviously had to see ki energy in action. And Shizuko had a plan.

Shizuko's plan was to propose to Dr Nakagawa that he should attempt to persuade a group of sympathetic, yet sceptical Europeans, that his methods worked. This, she told him, might lead to the BBC making a film about his work and dolphins. If this happened then the credibility of ki healing would be boosted world-wide.

Once the idea was seeded it quickly germinated. The outcome was that 12 people, including myself, Rebecca Fitzgerald and Stephen Rose, were invited to attend Nakagawa's clinic in Shimoda.

As a result of my previous experiences with Dr Nakagawa I felt there was a strong link between ki energy and dolphin healing. To explore it, I required a far greater understanding of ki and how it was used to treat patients with severe medical problems. The opportunity to visit Dr Nakagawa's treatment and training centre was just what I needed.

Our accommodation in Shimoda was typically Japanese. Bedding consisted of futons (mattresses) which were laid out on tatami matting on the floor each evening, and then rolled up and stored in cupboards during the day. The bedrooms were sparse; wash basins were in the corridor. Every morning there was a cleaning routine which nobody was excused. To me, it was an interesting expression of humility. Even places that looked meticulously clean were swept and dusted. Sticky tape was provided to deal with hairs and small specs of dust reluctant to leave their places of rest. I was told this ritual was not just an example of the Japanese obsession with cleanliness. It was a symbolic procedure, signifying that we were all equal – which no doubt we were in the eyes (if they had them) of any pathogenic bacteria or viruses lurking in the building.

Our accommodation, basic by our standards, was luxurious compared with that of the patients who set out their futons side by side each night in the same hall in which the healing sessions were held during the day.

The food, which was totally organic and vegetarian, was prepared with love and great joy by a noisy group from the countryside where the plants were grown on tiny plots, and carefully tended by hand. Each ingredient was selected for its special beneficial qualities.

Breakfast, after the early morning clean-up and an hour-long session of yoga-like exercise, was taken sitting on the floor beside low tables. It included miso soup, which was savoury and full of bits and pieces I didn't recognise. An optional extra with the soup were deep-red, salted dried plums, that I was told had good medicinal properties. These could be dropped into the soup or chewed like uncooked prunes.

Every day at Shimoda was packed with numerous therapeutic programmes taking place in different parts of the building. All of the participants were Japanese. We were invited to join any of these events and were provided with interpreters. We huddled around them as they told us what was going on in hushed tones.

At least once each day we all assembled in the main hall. We visitors sat on chairs in one corner. The Japanese sat, crosslegged, on the floor. These gatherings always incorporated a healing session in which everyone, ourselves included, sat or lay on the floor. As soon as the session started some of the audience would start writhing and making guttural sounds, noisily coughing out the 'guest energies' as Shizuko called them. This elimination of the causes of their medical problems was often accompanied by the secretion of saliva. Nakagawa's assistants stepped swiftly and deftly between them, performing mopping up operations with paper tissues. Some people groaned and moaned, some waved their arms, others rolled around. One patient's energy guest appeared to have a feline form. Every now and again the departing spirit would utter a loud 'meow'.

During these sessions all of the patients appeared to be in altered states of consciousness and completely unaware of what they were doing. Nakagawa walked amongst them channelling ki energy with his hands and always accompanied by the same continuously cascading music.

Immediately before these mass healing sessions, some of those assembled stood up, one at a time, and reported to

Dr Nakagawa and the rest of us what improvements in their medical condition had been made since the previous day. Dr Nakagawa listened to each one sympathetically and attentively. At the conclusion he commented, then gave advice and encouragement.

There is a Japanese belief that if more people took time out to enjoy a sunrise or a sunset there would be less violence in the world. I don't know if this thought was in the mind of the person who set the timetable, but one morning the entire group were driven in buses to the coast. Here we gathered on grassy banks facing the sea and meditated. We watched the sun in silence as it rose over the horizon and tinted with pink light the shimmering ocean dotted with small islands that was spread before us.

When Rebecca and I later reviewed the overall outcome of our visit to Shimoda I recalled how I had once been involved in a clinical trial to evaluate a new cough mixture. It was conducted in a hospital ward full of patients with chronic bronchitis. We strapped microphones to their throats and recorded on long play tapes how often they coughed before and after they received their medication. It was double blind, which meant that neither the patients nor the doctors knew which concoction contained the ingredient under investigation. Naturally we hoped, when all of the data were analysed, that our new wonder drug would be shown to have the cough-suppressing properties we were looking for. Rebecca and I agreed that there was absolutely no way we could remotely apply this kind of quantitative analysis to assess what happened in Shimoda.

Thoughts like this also caused me to change my mind about making a TV documentary. I could see no way of creating a balanced programme which, even with the most honourable of intentions and content, would not cause the cynics to pour scorn on what I had seen and experienced.

For me, the visit to Shimoda was immensely rewarding. It gave me a much better insight and understanding of a system of medicine that was very different from the one with which I was most familiar, ie the Western approach, in which specialisation was important and the saving and prolonging of life were the first priorities.

The visit also helped me to draw parallels between the work going on in Dr Nakagawa's clinic and the way in which dolphin healing seemed to work. I was convinced that Dr Nakagawa believed absolutely, and with utter sincerity, in what he was doing. His patients benefited from their treatment. He was offering hope, not immortality. In addition to ki, and inseparable from it, he gave his patients love and joy – a vital ingredient in dolphin healing. Dr Nakagawa and his patients accepted that they might die. Indeed, this happened when I revisited his treatment centre several years later. Just before I gave my presentation on dolphins one very seriously ill patient died. When the relatives came to take him away they said how pleased they were that he had been allowed to spend his last hours in the company of Dr Nakagawa. They said it had prepared him for the long journey ahead. Like many Japanese, they believed that their dear departed relative would eventually become a star in the heavens.

I recently heard an astrophysicist declare that there are more stars in the cosmos than grains of sand on the planet earth. So such a notion is not as numerically improbable as it might first appear! If one adds to this the ancient belief that dolphins carry the souls of the dead into the next world, then the prospect of death is transformed from sadness to pleasant anticipation.

Chapter 10
Dolphin Therapy Centres

In 1992 I was invited to open a new MIND centre based in an old converted printing works in Scunthorpe, Lincolnshire. MIND is a charity that helps those with mental problems, particularly depression. In the first instance it offers a sympathetic hearing and then advice in a non-threatening, welcoming environment, which is important for those whose self-esteem is at a low ebb. This is usually followed by counselling, often by people who have suffered similar problems themselves, and therefore know first hand the anguish that those needing help are going through. I was very impressed with what the organisation was doing and how it was setting about it.

After the opening ceremony was over an idea started to form in my mind. Could I take the MIND concept a stage further and incorporate dolphin healing into it? It was an ideal opportunity to apply what I call the Snowman Principle, which I define as follows:

Throw your concept, that is your snowman, up into the universe in the form of thought seeds. Snowflakes will form on these thought seeds. These snowflakes will then come fluttering down and settle themselves into a snowman. The snowman that finally creates itself is often different to the one you conceived in the first place. But it is invariably better.

My thought seeds on this occasion took the form of a publication which was distributed to the members of International Dolphin Watch and anyone else who cared to receive it. It was entitled *Dolphin Therapy Centres: A Vision for the Future*. The publication was in a bold blue cover, which was fortuitous because in its own way it had a similar role to that of a government blue paper which is a document for discussion. My blue paper opened with the following mission statement:

This report is not intended as a master plan, or to provide detailed proposals. Its aim is to outline the basic concept of Dolphin Therapy Centres (DTCs). By opening the idea for public debate it is hoped that even where DTCs themselves are not created perhaps some of the principles embodied in them will be incorporated in proposed therapy centres, or be introduced into existing establishments, where some of the ideas identified herein are already being practised.

This was followed by a summary:

Having established that encounters with dolphins can help people suffering from depression, it is proposed that DTCs should be set up. Captive dolphins will not be involved. Instead DTCs will accommodate pools in which the experience of meeting a dolphin in the sea will be artificially recreated. The dolphin therapy pool will be the focal point of every DTC. Counselling facilities and other complementary therapies will be available. Users of DTCs will also be encouraged to explore and develop their inherent artistic skills.

The DTCs will serve a multitude of purposes. One of them will be to help the ever-increasing number of people, estimated to be one in ten in Britain, who will need some form of psychiatric assistance during their lifetime. Another will be to reduce the stigma associated with mental distress. This will be achieved by helping sufferers regain their self-esteem and attain positions where they can be seen to contribute to society.

Any funds produced by the creative endeavours of those attending DTCs will be used to help dolphins.

A DTC will be a public manifestation of a tolerant and caring society which meets individual human needs and is concerned for the survival and welfare of other species.

By allying themselves with the dolphins, those suffering from mental distress will benefit from the spiritual energy of the dolphin which traditionally carries with it *hope, joy and love.*

The primary function of my proposed centres was to provide visitors with all the facilities necessary to overcome mental distress, and the problems that went with it. Having recovered their self-esteem I hoped they would find a way of re-integrating into normal community activities. I foresaw art as a major method of helping them get back on the rails. Thus the proposed centres would have facilities to enable visitors to develop whatever artistic talents they had. This would not be limited to painting. It would include writing, sculpture, dancing, music and even cooking, which I maintain can be both creative and artistic. The centres would provide a homely, cheerful, welcoming atmosphere. Each would incorporate a cafeteria, a recreation room, a library and a music/TV room, in addition to a counselling room – along lines similar to the MIND centre in Scunthorpe. Other rooms would be available for medical examinations and complementary therapies such as aromatherapy, reflexology, hypnotherapy, etc, as well as doubling as classrooms for art and drama. These would be attended by part-time art teachers, therapists and doctors.

DTCs would be friendly meeting places where those with mental problems could easily get help. With this in mind I proposed that they should be in urban areas where people normally congregate. I also felt that such centres should be based in old buildings to which those fallen on hard times could easily relate.

I felt that for some of those attending DTCs, engagement in various creative arts would be purely therapeutic. For others who had, or discovered they had, a real talent, and were able to develop it, then arrangements would be made for them to commercialise their work. Success in this and other activities raised what for me was an extremely important issue that would be absolutely fundamental to all DTCs. It was that we had to give something back to the dolphins, not just take from them. It was with this principle in mind that I proposed that income or funds raised should not just be used solely for helping humans. It should be deployed for helping dolphins also. Thus money raised would be directed towards providing wardens and information centres at places where direct interaction with dolphins in the wild was possible. At such locations visitors would learn about dolphins and be encouraged to treat them with respect. Monies would also be used for conservation projects, such as searching for methods of deterring whales and dolphins from drift nets and persuading fishermen to adopt a more tolerant and caring attitude towards cetaceans.

I wanted to set up a cycle in which *dolphins help people help dolphins*.

By embodying this concept of circulating dolphin energy, I hoped DTCs would help pave the path to a society in which humans would respect, care for and respond to the needs of all animals, as well as their fellows.

As soon as I mentioned DTCs, people immediately assumed I was talking about captive dolphins. So I had to make it absolutely clear that this was not so. All dolphins are entitled to a free life in their natural habitat. No dolphins would be captured and incarcerated in DTCs. The purpose of the proposed dolphin therapy pools was to recreate *artificially* the magic and joy of encounters with free dolphins who willingly choose to interact with humans in the open sea.

I pointed out in the report my own direct observations that swimming with dolphins appears to release profound emotional blocks. Dolphins make all of those who come into direct or indirect contact with them feel special in some way. Dolphins seemed somehow to restore self-esteem and self-confidence. To me this was perhaps their most powerful contribution in helping those suffering from depression. Another observation I made was that everyone responded differently to dolphins, and that dolphin-linked steps to recovery were made in association with other treatments. Thus at DTCs dolphin therapy would be combined with conventional and/or complementary treatments, thereby enabling those seeking help to find the most appropriate combination for their own personality and needs.

Finally, I suggested that it was highly likely that ancient civilisations knew that dolphins benefited humans. Although DTCs were a new concept, all I was doing was rediscovering what was already known in bygone years and by aboriginal people. Having thrown my thought seeds up into the universe in the form of an IDW publication, I reckoned it would be at least ten years before the snowman eventually formed.

On this score, I was totally wrong.

Chapter 11
The Dolphin Healing Centre

It was Shizuko and Dr Nakagawa who were responsible for my getting the anticipated time-scale for the introduction of Dolphin Therapy Centres completely wrong. When it happened in 1992, less than a year after I published the proposal, I realised that the concept of dolphin healing, which I thought would take years to permeate into human consciousness, was accelerating like a racing car. When it happened so quickly I pondered on which mysterious forces, that I didn't know about, were at work.

At the time I published my blue paper, Dr Nakagawa's techniques were being adopted widely in Japan. One of those who decided to develop their application was Kokyo Ishizaki, a priest responsible for the Gyokuryuin which was part of the Myoren-ji Temple founded in 1294 in Kyoto, the old capital of Japan.

In the early post-war years, the temple was at the centre of a tight local community. Then, just as in Britain and elsewhere, rapid socio-economic changes took place. These led to a shift in the number of children born in each family as well as a decline in attendance at the temple. One outcome of this was that the kindergarten at the Gyokuryuin, which was run by the priest's wife, Konoe, was closed.

Kokyo and Konoe had three children. One of their daughters, Aiko, as well as Konoe herself, was subject to bouts of depression. In addition Konoe had a form of multiple sclerosis (MS) which affected her co-ordination and made her unsteady on her feet. Konoe responded well to Nakagawa's ki energy treatment. She was not cured, but her condition improved. As a result two of Nakagawa's Hi Genki machines were installed in the kindergarten and were made available to anyone attending the temple.

Not long after I touched her 'dolphin button', as she put it, Shizuko visited the temple and touched the priest's button. When she did so she was unwittingly tapping into a long tradition amongst the Buddhists of Japan, who have always had a special reverence for the cetaceans. In earlier times if a whale stranded and died, the priest would conduct a special ceremony on the shore to ensure that the spirit of the whale was safely returned to the oceans.

This spiritual connection was kept alive in Japan by a thread, despite the attitude that prevailed throughout the rest of the world for over a century in which whales were regarded as an unlimited resource to be exploited by humans.

The extent of the whale-hunting industry – and dolphins are small whales – is no more poignantly told than in Heathcote Williams' epic illustrated poem, *Whale Nation*. At the end of this immensely moving evocation the poet reveals:

In the Koganji Temple in Yamaguchi Province
Tombs have been built to dead whales.
The monuments are facing the sea;
Thus, it is thought, the whales may pay homage to
    their dead.
The inscription on one reads:

'You whales who have perished,
Although you cannot return to the world,
We will cherish your memory long in our hearts.
In Arikawara there is a memorial to six hundred
    whales;
In the Chudoji Temple of Muroto, there is a shrine for
    a thousand.
Each year in Yamaguchi, a ceremony is conducted
In memory of the souls of the unborn,
And to lift a curse on man for killing so many whales.

After I published my proposal I never gave the remotest thought to the possibility that a Dolphin Therapy Centre should come into existence in Japan. However, in hindsight, putting ki and the Buddhist tradition together makes sense. When Shizuko passed the thought seed to the priest and his wife it germinated rapidly.

In November 1993 Rebecca, Shizuko and I, with many others, presided over the official opening of the Ki and Dolphin Healing Centre.

The hall where the children once gathered and played was the size of a large classroom. It was directly connected to the living quarters of the priest and his family. We all stayed in a hostel which was part of the Temple complex. It provided basic accommodation for pilgrims and visitors. We were each given a small bowl, a tiny towel and a bar of soap to use when we visited the public bath- and wash-house a few streets away. The passage to the bedrooms passed beside the Rock Garden of Sixteen Arhyats. It was a typical Japanese stylised garden complete with trickling water feature – a place of great tranquillity for quiet relaxation and contemplation.

As is customary in all Japanese dwellings, we left our street shoes in cubicles at the entrance and stepped into loose slippers. The temple had many treasures, including 42 panels of calligraphy and masterpieces of the Hasegawa school of screen painting. These paintings of manicured trees and distant mountains were kept in rooms that we passed on the way to the dormitories.

Dolphin Healing

Before the opening ceremony I attended the early morning service in the nearby Prayer Hall. Entering it was like going into a vast treasure-filled church bedecked with magnificent hangings. Rich yellow light from guttering candles reflected off ornate gilded fittings. It was full of mystery.

The service itself was conducted with solemnity by the robed priest. The ancient ceremony with its chanting, and deep resonating sounds issuing from a huge brass gong, struck with a heavy wooden hammer, seemed to touch long forgotten memories. Deep inside me the sharp edges of reality diffused into another space. For a time I transcended into a world beyond my earthly existence.

The Ki and Dolphin Healing Centre was separated from the Prayer Hall where religious services were conducted. The large single room had an atmosphere all of its own that was completely different. The walls of the Dolphin Healing Centre were decorated with pictures of dolphins. It was peaceful, but there was a vibrancy about the place which connected it to the here and now. The Prayer Hall took care of the soul. The Gyokuryuin part of the temple complex looked after the mind.

One of the first people who had come there for help before the official opening was a deaf and dumb woman, whose husband had left her and whose 14-year-old son had become violent and anti-social. She was severely depressed and expressed her problem in writing to Shizuko. Somehow Shizuko picked up the essence of sign language and soon exchanges were taking place with gesticulating arms. Japanese characters, written at incredible speed on pieces of paper, quickly littered the floor on which they sat. It rapidly became clear that the problem was not just that of the mother. The son needed help as well.

The son, a surly individual, arrived with his mother for the opening ceremony that evening. As time passed it was interesting to note the gradual changes that came over him. At first he refused to participate at all. By the end of the evening he diffidently joined in the general jollity. Up to that time he vigorously refuted that he had any need of help. When he left he agreed to return at a later date with his mother for ki treatment and dolphin healing by the priest and his wife.

The mother and son would not be able to experience dolphin healing in a pool, one of the key ingredients of my DTC vision, for the very obvious reason that there wasn't one. But they would be in a healing environment in which I hoped they would find ground on which to bring into the open the deeply emotional issues which we felt were at the seat of both of their mental problems. Because the mother was deaf and dumb they were compelled to communicate via writing and sign language. I wondered if, with care and understanding, these exchanges could be adapted into painting and dance forms. Could art help to bridge the chasm that had formed between the son and his mother? Even if it was wishful thinking, I felt that by agreeing to come back at least the first step towards a healing process had been made.

After the opening ceremony public meetings were held at the centre which were advertised in the local press. These were most often focused on the presence of a visitor, such as Shizuko, who would make a presentation to the gathering. In between times, clients would come for individual counselling and treatments.

The Ki and Dolphin Healing Centre also became a repository for dolphin music and art from around the world, linking the past traditions with the present. The priest, who himself was very artistic, designed an emblem in the form of two kissing dolphins whose silhouettes enclosed a heart-shaped space. One dolphin had its mouth open. The other had its mouth closed. These symbolically represented the yin and yang dogs that are placed at the entrance to many Shinto shrines to ward off evil spirits. You'll have noticed the emblem at the start of each chapter.

Staying at the Dolphin Centre in Kyoto gave visitors like me an insight into the Japanese psyche that I would never have gained as a tourist. Shizuko also introduced me to other aspects of Japanese culture that helped me understand more fully how it was that ki and dolphin healing had found acceptance in the country that I, as an ignorant Westerner, would have least expected.

Shizuko took us to visit two of her brothers, missioners at the new Shinto-based order of Oomoto, near Kyoto.

The Oomoto faith, which had two million followers in pre-war Japan, was founded in 1892 by Nao Deguchi, an illiterate, middle-aged country woman who was told to write down, with automatic writing, what an inner voice had to say. The message began: 'The Greater world shall burst into bloom as plum blossoms at winter's end.' What she was predicting was that the time was imminent for the entire world to move into a new age of love and harmony. The person whose mission was to help her fulfil this prophecy was an extraordinary man, Onisaburo Deguchi, who amongst many other achievements wrote 81 volumes of scripture. Onisaburo maintained that all religions stemmed from one divine God. In 1925 he established the Jinrui Aizenkai, or ULBA (Universal Love and Brotherhood Association) to bring together all religions in an attempt to induce all members of the human race to love one another and establish eternal peace.

This ideal ran contrary to government policy in a country that was preparing for war. In 1936 most of Oomoto's buildings and sanctuaries were dynamited. Nonetheless the ideal lived on. After the war it was left to the third spiritual leader of Oomoto, Madame Naohi Deguchi, to carry the ideal forward. She recognised the immense value of her father's art. At the instigation of Shizuko's husband, Kees Ouwehand, an exhibition *The Art of Onisaburo Deguchi and His School* was opened in Paris in 1972. From there it went around Europe to North America, the last showing being in San Francisco in 1975.

It was James Morton, Dean of the cathedral in New York City, who first used the term 'New Age' to describe different religions working harmoniously together. It started when he allowed Kyotaro Deguchi, son of Madame Naohi Deguchi, who was touring with the art exhibition, to perform a Shinto ceremony in his cathedral.

Finally, in 1992, Naohi Deguchi was able to bring her dream

of a building in Oomoto in which all religions could come together to worship into reality. At its opening, the Hall of Immortality (Choseiden) as it was called, was filled with religious dignitaries from around the world.

It was not long after this that the group of us who had gathered at Shimoda to learn about ki were taken and shown the ruins of the old buildings and invited to say a prayer and participate in religious ceremonies in the new Hall of Immortality at Oomoto. We were also introduced to the delicate intricacies of the traditional Japanese tea ceremony.

When we came away we could certainly identify better how it was that the Japanese were able to take on board new concepts like dolphin healing and not see it as incompatible with long-held beliefs and traditions. Up until my visits to Shimoda, Kyoto and Oomoto I had regarded the Japanese as the arch consumers, which indeed they were. In Japan the national ethic was: produce, use and trash in quick order. Little or no regard was paid to conservation. After my visit I was aware that the Japanese were capable of profound change, and that change was under way.

Two years later Shizuko and I were invited by the mayor of Hitachi to give a presentation at a huge public entertainment event. Hitachi is a city that has grown rich on the production of consumer goods. When we were dining together the mayor confided in me that he hadn't really wanted to stand for office because he thought his views on conservation and moving to a more caring, spiritual society were far too radical in a city founded on ever-expanding consumerism. Yet much to his surprise he was elected with an overwhelming majority. He had a special concern for physically and mentally handicapped people. He invited us because he had heard of the Ki and Dolphin Healing Centre in Kyoto.

At the end of our presentation in Hitachi, the priest, his wife and daughter came up on to the stage. Hastily duplicated copies of The Dolphin Song, *Iruka No Uta*, written by Konoe Ishizaki for the opening ceremony of the Ki and Dolphin Healing Centre, had been distributed to the packed crowd in the immense auditorium. The audience, led by Shizuko, sang along to a song about dolphin love. At the same time, in a spectacular laser display, whales and dolphins danced on the wall at the back of the stage. Reflecting on it afterwards made me wonder if it would be the Japanese, and not the British, Germans or Americans, who would lead the world towards more spiritual values, which I foresee as the next major phase in the evolution of our civilisation.

Chapter 12
Exploring Autism

By 1996 I felt the time had come for those interested in dolphin therapy to have a serious seminar. With the aid of Kath Huddlestone of the Spiritual Venturers Association, a Dolphin Healing Conference was organised in London. Its aim was to gather together people working on different aspects of dolphin healing, to exchange ideas, and project into the future.

The event took place at Regent's Park College in the heart of London on 30 June 1996. Delegates trekked in from around the world. Almost all of those attending had had personal crises that dolphins had helped them come to terms with. There was laughter, there were tears. It was an emotional experience for everyone present, more intense for some than others. Being totally objective was virtually impossible, emphasising yet again how difficult it is to separate science and magic when dealing with dolphins. Dr Olivia de Bergerac and William MacDougal, co-founders of the Dolphin Within Society (now the Dolphin Society) in Australia contributed a scientific element. Using the latest technology they skilfully blended slides and videos. They showed the changes in brain patterns that followed when stressed-out, hard-nosed businessmen were persuaded by

Olivia, a psychotherapist, to become like children and frolic with dolphins in the sea.

Kokyo and Konoe Ishizaki, the priest and his wife, came to England for the first time to attend the conference. The priest, with immense dignity and dressed in his traditional robes, told of many remarkable healings that had taken place at the Dolphin Healing Centre. With Shizuko translating, he explained that the divine spirit was present in all things, animal, vegetable and mineral. Everyone had powers to heal. Dolphins, he said, released this energy and enabled it to flow freely through humans, thereby helping to restore their health. Music and art added to this process. He totally captivated the audience. Several commented to me afterwards that Kokyo himself radiated a powerful feeling of strength and peace that in itself was healing.

One of the delegates, who was well known to the Ishizakis, was Lilo Slumiok Müller from Germany. When she was diagnosed as having terminal cancer Lilo refused to give in to the disease. She scoured the world looking for treatments. Her search took her to Japan where she met Dr Nakagawa and Shizuko. After that she and Shizuko became companions. Dolphins, coupled with ki energy administered by Dr Nakagawa, helped her to overcome the disease. The surgeons who predicted her imminent death opened her up when she pronounced herself cured. To their surprise and disbelief they found that all of the tumours, which had proliferated throughout Lilo's body, had disappeared. Her cancer regressed completely and she became a ki healer in her own right.

Lilo was an extraordinary woman in more ways than one. She discovered she was psychic at an early age, a characteristic inherited from her grandmother. Internal investigation of the source of severe abdominal pain when she was 21 revealed that some of her organs were duplicated. She had three kidneys, two stomachs and two uteruses. These were not apparent from her external appearance and did not stop her giving birth to two girls. It did, however, result in her having to undergo a number of operations. During several of those she described how she left her body and watched the surgeons performing their procedures.

From her stylishly coiffed silver-grey hair I guessed she might have been in her fifties, but her age was hard to tell because she was always impeccably dressed and made up. I never saw her look anything but immaculate – even when she had just come out of the water on a Dolphinswim trip in the Bahamas.

Being on board a boat with Lilo for a week gave me an opportunity to get to know her. Lilo usually carried coloured pencils and pens with her to illustrate points she wished to make. When I asked her how she thought dolphins were helping her, she drew a series of rainbow-coloured pictures. Through these she explained how the dolphins took her aura (energy bands surrounding her physical body), cleansed it, and then returned it to her.

At the conference I reported on how I had set up Operation Sunflower ten years earlier and how it had evolved into an ongoing research project. The meeting itself was evidence that the ramifications of dolphin healing were expanding like the rings from a pebble dropped into a pond. Two of the first major participants, whose case histories convinced me that the mysterious therapeutic power of dolphins was worth exploring, were present. They each gave accounts of their personal encounters with dolphins in the sea and how these experiences completely changed their lives.

Bill Bowell was there with his wife, Edna, who he referred to as his 'land dolphin' because of her selfless support throughout his 11 years of darkness with chronic depression. He explained what it was like to live in what he described as a mental black hole, and how none of the treatments offered by the best medical brains in Oxford had helped. Most of the audience were in tears when he described how, when swimming with Simo the dolphin off the coast of Wales, a glimmer of light appeared in his darkness. It revealed an escape route out of the torment of depression. Bill had followed it and was now completely in the light once again.

Bill was reunited with Jemima Biggs, a fellow guinea pig. With baby Phoebe on her hip she explained how she had moved from near death with anorexia nervosa to becoming a mother after joining Bill to swim with Fungie off the coast of Dingle.

All these speakers helped to pull together and highlight the powerful evidence for dolphin healing in their own lives.

The baffling mental condition of autism was also high on the agenda. Autism crosses all race boundaries and is estimated to affect one in 2000 of the entire human population. The symptoms and severity vary widely. Virtually every case is different. In the movie *The Rain Man*, Dustin Hoffman plays the role of an autistic man who is obsessed with routine. He appears to be an idiot, yet has a remarkable memory, which his brother tries to use to his advantage in casinos.

Stephen Wiltshire is an autist with exceptional gifts. He has an ability to memorise immensely complex architecture – even city scapes – with total accuracy. Stephen's genius has found an outlet in art. His line drawings have been heralded as masterpieces, and several books of his work have been published. Despite the fact that he has a speech impediment, and finds it hard to communicate verbally, he has perfect pitch and can identify the notes of any chord on an analytical level that some experts have compared to the genius of Mozart. Yet, despite his fame, his fortune, and intensive attention by his mother and others, Stephen's social skills are extremely limited. He doesn't play sport because he has no idea what winning or losing means. The value of money means absolutely nothing to him.

One of the most characteristic features of those classified as autistic is that they do not show emotional responses apart from frustration. Thus they appear to be cocooned in their own worlds where they cannot be reached. Perhaps the most disturbing of all is that they appear to be empty of love. But are they? Is what we see as their problem not an inability to feel emotions, but rather an inability to express them?

For most people autism is a very distressing condition. Some autists also have fits. Many clever minds have been applied to analysing the condition, to bring autists into the world which the rest of us regard as normal, and therefore desirable. This was the case with Eve Hanf-Enos who was scheduled to give a presentation with her mother Brigitte during the afternoon of our conference. Her story is extraordinary.

Eve was born by Caesarean section on 28 September 1971 of two highly intelligent parents, one a professor of mathematics at Oxford University, the other a very talented artist. The symptoms of Eve's autism were not apparent until she was a year old, at which time her mother and father went away on a business trip for seven weeks, leaving Eve in the care of her grandparents. When her parents returned, Eve's mother, Brigitte, noticed that her child was showing obsessive behaviour, constantly turning a leaf around in her hands. Eve did not develop like other children.

When her parents divorced, Eve went to live with her mother in a house close to that of her maternal grandparents in the US. Shortly after she arrived, Eve's grandparents split up. Her grandfather went back to his homeland, Germany. As a consequence Eve was looked after by her mother and grandmother, Lotte Hanf. Eve never gained any of the social graces of other children. She could barely feed herself, and could not, or did not want to control her bowels voluntarily. She needed supervision around the clock. Eve was, however, a stunningly beautiful child, with dark hair, cherry red lips and a porcelain complexion. Her looks remained compellingly attractive, although slightly disfigured, after she smashed her face into a drinking glass during a fit. The glass shattered and lacerated her face, leaving scars close to her lips.

Eve was diagnosed as autistic; the cause was unknown. Apart from medication for her fits, the medical profession was at a loss to prescribe curative treatment. Eve showed no emotional response, no matter how much affection was lavished upon her. The stress on Eve's mother, who continued to pursue her career as an artist, was enormous. Brigitte explored every avenue she could to bring her child out of autism. One of those whose help she sought was Patricia St John, a member of the

International Marine Animal Trainers' Association and a specialist in non-verbal communication, especially between humans and dolphins. Patricia had observed that some aspects of dolphin behaviour in captivity were similar to those of autistic children. Patricia was convinced that dolphins and children with autism could transmit their thoughts to her directly, without going through language. When Eve and her mother visited Patricia at her home in Connecticut, Patricia sensed that Eve was distressed at finding herself in unfamiliar surroundings, especially with dogs bounding around. She remembered that the dolphins she had swam with in a pool were more willing to interact with her when she adopted a submissive attitude. So Patricia did the same thing with Eve. She curled up on the floor in a non-threatening position. And it worked. Eve's tension started to ease. Then Eve used her hands to draw Patricia's face towards her. Eve planted her lips firmly on Patricia's. In that brief moment Patricia felt that an exchange was taking place that was similar to the exploration dolphins made, with their sonar.

In order to explore her theories on different methods of communication, Patricia needed to work with autistic children and dolphins, and so she visited Eve at home. During one of these visits, Brigitte made an important discovery.

'They say there's nothing wrong with you – show me,' Brigitte exploded in a rage of despair at Eve. She pushed a pen into Eve's fingers and supported her hand.

'What's your name? Write.'

Instead of the endless circles and scribbles which were usually produced, the letters EVE slowly appeared.

From that time on Eve and Brigitte jointly developed what was called facilitated communication. Brigitte would support Eve's limp finger to enable her to type out words on a keyboard.

When Eve started to write in this way Brigitte learnt that her daughter had taught herself to read, and that one of her favourite authors was Dostoevsky. Brigitte was unaware of Eve's love of literature until she found out, via Eve's halting, palsied print, that she had been sneaking out of her room at night and taking books from the shelf. As the months went by Eve's writing ability improved dramatically. So did its contents. Her poetry was astounding. As Eve emerged at the age of 14, from a gamine, doll-like child to a fully fledged adolescent her frustrations, her desires, her angers and her demands poured forth. But Eve still refused to speak.

In 1985 Brigitte and Patricia took Eve to Sealand at Cape Cod, a dolphinarium where Patricia had communicated with a captive dolphin named Scotty. Eve hated seeing Scotty incarcerated and later wrote a powerful poem expressing her anger and sadness. Despite this, in 1990, she agreed to go back to the dolphinarium, this time to swim with Scotty.

Eve was terrified of going in the water. Gradually Patricia won her over, telling Eve she didn't have to go in unless she wanted to. Eventually Eve went into a pool of very warm water, but it was obvious that going into the cold water of the dolphinarium was more than she could take. Eve and her mother stood by the dolphin pool and played ball with Scotty. Then the dolphin got bored. For a moment he stopped in front of Eve and the two stared at one another. A moment later the trainer arrived with a bucket of fish. Contact was broken, but Patricia was absolutely convinced that Eve and Scotty had communicated, Brigitte then took Eve away to the ladies' room. And there, for Brigitte's ears only, Eve uttered her first word 'Good'. Brigitte was hoping this was the beginning of a breakthrough and that Eve would begin to speak. But Eve wouldn't utter another word, no matter how much she was coaxed. Nonetheless, the fact that she had spoken a word, instead of grunting, made Brigitte even more resolved to find a solution to her daughter's problems.

When a conference to explore unexplained phenomena was proposed, Brigitte offered to make a contribution on autism and facilitated writing. The event duly took place in Santa Fé, New Mexico in 1993.

Ki energy healing came under the remit of the Santa Fé conference, and Dr Nakagawa was invited to attend with

Shizuko acting as his interpreter. Prior to the conference, Shizuko had become friendly with the Ishizaki family who had attended several of Dr Nakagawa's seminars at Shimoda. One of the reasons for their presence was to seek help for one of their daughters, Utako, who had a nervous skin problem, neurodermatitis. During a healing session it became apparent that Utako had several 'guest energies'. Shizuko later visited Utako to give her ki healing at her temple home at Gyokuryuin. During the session Shizuko invited Utako's guest energies to leave. One of them appeared to be a former street boy, who spoke directly to Shizuko via Utako, who uttered his words with a deep male voice in a Kyoto dialect. If Shizuko had told me this story before I went to Shimoda and witnessed for myself what happened to people under the influence of ki, I would have found it impossible to believe. But as she recounted the incident I could picture the scene exactly as Shizuko described it.

The street boy told Shizuko there were lots more like him inside Utako.

'Then how do I persuade you all to go?' asked Shizuko.

'Sing to us,' he responded.

As it happened Shizuko had been receiving singing lessons from an opera singer. So she started to sing to channel or transmit her ki/dolphin healing energy by singing an aria.

'No, no, not like that,' screamed the boy. 'That singing is full of ego. Just do it with a sweet voice.'

He then demonstrated; a gentle, lilting sound coming from Utako's lips. Shizuko imitated him.

'That's better.'

And so Shizuko started singing to Utako as the street boy had taught her.

'Thank you,' said the street boy. 'Now I can float away like a feather on the wind.' And he was gone. Shizuko finished her treatment. When Utako came back into full consciousness she shook herself. The weight that had been pressing on her mind was no longer there. She felt much better.

With this experience still clearly in her mind Shizuko

encountered Eve, sitting on her own in a corridor, at the conference in Santa Fé.

Again, because I had seen it myself many times, I could envisage what happened next when Shizuko related it to me much later.

Shizuko got permission to sit beside Eve from her mother. Then, quite spontaneously, she started to treat Eve with ki energy by singing. Eve responded with a staring look. She took Shizuko's head between her hands, their lips touched. Shizuko's face was covered with Eve's saliva. Shizuko perceived that a channel was open. With her lips close to Eve's, Shizuko started to sing into Eve's partly open mouth, just as the street boy had told her.

'Then Eve wanted to look into my mouth deeply. So I sang with my mouth as widely open as possible.' Eve pointed and stuck her lips into Shizuko's mouth.

'It was so beautiful,' Shizuko told me. 'Eve was drinking healing energy through me. I was feeding her with musical sounds like a blackbird feeding its young.'

Eve stared back at Shizuko. Eve wasn't looking *at* Shizuko, she was looking *into* Shizuko. Shizuko felt she was being invited to swim in Eve's eyes.

'It was a very dark and quiet place there, like a mountain lake,' she told me. Shizuko then reciprocated.

'Come and swim into my eyes now like a dolphin,' cooed Shizuko as she continued to hum, and then sing the song 'Oh what a beautiful morning'.

Eve again pressed her lips to Shizuko's and gazed steadfastly into her eyes. As she told me the story, Shizuko was reliving the moment. 'I had never experienced anything like it before.' Tears filled Shizuko's eyes as she continued singing to me, demonstrating how she had sung to Eve.

And that was how Brigitte met Shizuko for the first time. Eve and Shizuko were lost together in each other's eyes. Shizuko was singing softly, her face covered with Eve's slobber. It was then that Eve articulated the word 'Good', loudly and distinctly, not just for her mother to hear, but Shizuko as well.

When Shizuko heard this she knew that Eve could speak properly if she wanted to.

Their common connection with dolphins was a cement that bonded Eve, Shizuko and Brigitte together instantly. When they later heard Rebecca Fitzgerald, who was also in Santa Fé, talk about her work with dolphins, it seemed as if destiny had laid out a path in front of Eve. All she had to do now was follow it. And, with Shizuko acting as pathfinder, it led eventually to me.

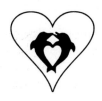

Chapter 13
Eve in Amsterdam

Shizuko felt sure that dolphins held the key to solving Eve's problems and was prepared to travel to the US to help. Shizuko kept me updated on her visits to Eve's home in Connecticut. A stream of drawings, letters and poems started to drop through my letter box. Included among them was a book of poems by Eve and an earlier manuscript for a short autobiographical book, completed in 1989, entitled *I am a Hypothesis* by Eve Hanf-Enos and Brigitte Hanf. It was an amazing, heartrending story, and started with a quote:

> It was the failures who had always won, but by the time they won they had come to be called successes. This is the final paradox, which men call evolution.
>
> [Loren Eiseley, quoted in *I am a Hypothesis*
> by Eve Hanf-Enos and Brigitte Hanf,
> private publication, 1989]

Then, like a fibre-optic inspection of a faulty heart, it probed the recesses of the authors' minds. It revealed the anguish of

Brigitte's relationship with her father and a disturbing account of a past-life experience:

> A year ago, in a period of intense disturbance fraught with seizures, Eve described her previous existence as an inmate in a concentration camp. She had tried to escape with her half-starved brother on her back (in this life she is an only child), but was caught and thrown back into the gas oven on to a heap of burning bodies.

Eve's facilitated writing advanced to the use of a small keyboard which she referred to as a 'hip machine' because it would fit into a hip pocket. This considerably increased the speed and readability of her writings.

In August 1994 Shizuko and her friend Sumine Hayashibara, a classical violinist, visited Eve and her mother at their home in Connecticut.

'When I first met her I was frightened because her body movements were so violent at times,' Sumine later told me. 'It was like confronting an angry animal. I didn't know what to do. But when I saw Shizuko communicating with Eve my fears gradually subsided. Eve seems to be able to see inside my head – that too is a bit scary,' Sumine added. 'People tend to treat her like a child and she doesn't like that.'

Sumine took a gift for Eve, a violin, and played 'Ave Maria' on it. Eve showed violent frustration. 'I want to play like that and I cannot,' said Eve's keyboard.

Shizuko was somebody Eve could easily communicate with. Soon the two were exchanging messages. Eve confided her hopes and fears to Shizuko.

'I want to pop out of autism,' came up on the VDU of Eve's computer. 'But I feel oppositional. I am afraid I will be very lonely afterwards.'

Shizuko discovered that Eve was a gifted writer. 'She has an immense joy of word play, often creating her own words,' Shizuko told me. 'Sometimes she can control a pencil sufficiently to draw. I feel she could break out of her autism. But how? I think in Eve's mind her autism makes her a special person. She doesn't want to lose that specialness.'

When Shizuko gave Eve a copy of *Dilo and the Call of the Deep*, a children's book I had written about a dolphin named Dilo, Eve assimilated the story immediately. She clung on to the book fiercely. She took it to bed with her. The next day, via her hip machine, Shizuko discovered that Eve remembered every word in the book. 'I felt Eve somehow identified with Dilo. Perhaps it was because Dilo is a special dolphin. Because she is autistic, Eve is a special person.'

Shizuko felt that Eve needed a task. She suggested to Eve that she could lead a group to help other autistic people. To everyone's surprise Eve wrote 'Wow. I accept it,' and agreed to become president. Eve then typed up the words – Dilo Group.

'What will you do as President of the Dilo Group?' asked Shizuko. The answer came back instantly on the keyboard. 'I would like to give a gift of joy and laughter to other sad people . . . I don't know how . . . I feel groups should be about humour and dipping into mind ideas,' commented Eve.

Shizuko told me, 'Eve has a great talent for leading people. She has an insight into the heads of other people. I feel she has a role to play in helping other autistic people. By doing that she will find the courage she needs to come out of her own autism. Eve loves music, she loves dolphins and she loves Dilo. They all have a role to play.'

Shizuko's idea that giving Eve a task would open a route for her to the outside world was effective. Eve's presidency of the Dilo Group inspired a torrent of words to pour from her computer. In January 1995 I received the following letter from Eve.

4 January 1995
(*Transcribed from Eve's communicator*)

An open letter to Dilo members and all lovers of our fellow swimmers in the ocean of life.

Opinion I have that isolated people all over the globe are stopping for taking a look around in whichever place they find themselves. I safely wanted to live all my life. Opinions I opposed of anyone who lopped me off from security. Time or place were irrelevant. I only lots of protection wanted and to be looked after in comfort. Oppositional I felt to popping into life. A happy day came when I lifted my silence in written words. Soon I popped out in other ways like enjoying meeting people on their turf and willingly leaving my warm hole to risk the winds of change. In time people lost their fear of my looniness and opened possibilities of friendship. Possibilities of love and laughter began to emerge and I found I loved laughing and music . . .

The poem we send you was written after the encounter with Scotty the dolphin I mentioned earlier. Dominating my memory down the several years since I met him, he opened my life. Pining over his lost life I try to remind myself of the question we all ask: if we live or if we don't live our lives, we are responsible for our deaths? What I mean is, to what are we owing the powers that shape us? Do we shape ourselves or are we shaped by energies we are not able to recognise yet? Or both? Or neither? My feeling is options we are given throughout our lives and our job is to learn to recognise and act on them. This we learned especially. Piling up options over the years, we refused to see them, let alone act on them. Isolated from my own needs my life was as murky as Scotty's prison. One day he raised himself into the light. One day I did too, but I want to live in light having found it, and Scotty couldn't.

Dilo people need to raise ourselves above the dark stagnant parts of our lives. They are probably safe places but we must jettison our lifejackets if we are to swim.

I am looking forward to meeting you.

Love, Eve

However, it was in the poem that accompanied this letter that Eve better exposed some of the thoughts which were occupying her mind. The way in which she expressed her feelings about Scotty, the dolphin who had caused her to say her first word, moved me deeply.

Martyr

Tumbling wild through manmade murk
Trawling balls of colored hell
Tightwound by endless boundaries
Of demands, rewards, applause
A mortal creature, terrible in his torture
Beauty sold to mobs of vacationed boredom
Themselves mortal creatures imprisoned
In knotted webs of their own making
I dared to scream my rage
Yell my heart's despair
At misery measured in balls and hoops
Thrown to shouts and bungled music
To win men's mammon
I fled

Only must and I did return
To the silent stinking pooled prison
Alone after all
I weeping waited
Death alone could be so still
I waited
With imploding heartbeats
I waited

Exploding his streaming metal sheening shape
From its water hell
Impossibly end upright in perfect balance on his fanning fin
During an eon's time he held me in his eye

And I held him
Each in each and one together
Magnified in time and love
We flew through seas of light and life
Then back he sank
And so did I
I spoke one word, my mute mouth cried
'Good!'

The next year the dolphin died.

[Eve Hanf-Enos]
January 1995

Shizuko wanted to introduce Eve and Brigitte to some of her friends and contacts who she thought might accelerate Eve's journey out of autism. She persuaded Eve and her mother to travel to the Netherlands where she had arranged a Dolphins' Poetry and Autism Afternoon for Sunday 13 May 1995 at OIBIBIO, a cafe and spiritual centre in the heart of Amsterdam, close to the railway station. I was scheduled to give a film show at a divers' conference in Rotterdam on 12 May, and could remain in Holland for an extra day. The time had come for me to meet Eve, which I did in Amsterdam.

There was no form to the Dolphins' Poetry and Autism meeting. It just flowed in a very magical way. Eve sat at a table with Shizuko and her mother facing the audience of about 40 people in a large room. Eve was armed with her hip machine via which she communicated with the audience, with the aid of her mother who supported Eve's index finger as it tapped the keys and then read out the words as they appeared on the display panel.

After reading out a poem entitled 'I am who we are', written by Eve in January 1994, Brigitte made reference to Eve's 'doppelgänger existence'. By this she was referring to the two Eves. There was the one that everybody could see – an attractive woman, who looked younger than her years, whose unsmiling gaze was constantly wandering, often towards the ceiling, who although sitting in front of us appeared to be lost in her own dream world. The other was the inner Eve, the literate poet and essayist whose only way of communicating was via her keyboard.

The poem concluded with the powerful lines:

I am who we are
Separated by this bagged body and united by one soul
Each of us alone, and all made a whole.

I felt however that perhaps a triplegänger (if such a word exists) existence would perhaps have been more appropriate because Brigitte was an integral part of Eve's life. Like other sceptics of facilitated writing I wondered how many of the words attributed to Eve were from her mother who was guiding the hand with the limp finger that was tapping out the letters on the keyboard. Shizuko was absolutely convinced that the words were purely Eve's. Fascinating exchanges took place, via the keyboard between Eve and her audience. The subject of non-verbal communication was discussed. One woman who was obviously at an advanced stage of pregnancy felt that Eve was communicating directly with her unborn child.

Everyone, including myself, deemed the afternoon a great success.

A short time after this, my first meeting with Eve, I received a very positive letter from Connecticut. It was Eve's second open letter to the Dilo group.

1 June 1995

Pending my imminent lipwords I must once more
resort to printed words. Glad I feel in knowing you in
a new way now that we've met and seen who we all
are. Hollering yahoo I option take since our kopping
out of kopping out session in Amsterdam. Past worries
are fast receding into the distance as I'm learning to use
the new tools you've given me. If you are still as close

in thought in a year or two I'll be in fantastic form.
Jolly good Horace really got us off to a piping hot start.

Rats run in mazes in cages and people run mazes in
their heads and both get lost until they find hope in the
shape of fellow maze runners who know their way. For
some of you dolphins play the leading role in helping
you find the way out. For me who hasn't swum yet
with a dolphin, you have quietly caused a revolution in
my head – it's OK to get lost because you will always
be found. Easy to say and not nearly as hard to do as I
thought.

Good friends come in disguises more often than we
know and in Amsterdam I met many. Dolphins brought
us together and will keep us together. Thank you again
and again for daring me to come. For now, we must lop
off written words but you will dread the day when you
won't be able to shut me up.

Love, Eve

'Lipwords' was Eve's way of referring to speech. 'Lop off' was
her way of saying 'stop'. The last sentence of her letter implied
that she was preparing to start talking. It seemed that her desire
to break out of autism was well under way.

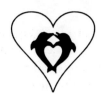

Chapter 14
Panama City Beach

We all felt the next step for Eve's development was to meet a dolphin in the open sea. But where and in what circumstances? Finances were limited.

The answer turned out to be Panama City Beach in Florida where a Belgian, Michel Atlas, had set up the Human Dolphin Institute. The institute was a place where people could go to meet and be healed by dolphins whilst maintaining the highest ethical standards from the human and dolphin points of view. Visitors were encouraged to think in terms of the total ecology of the area, not just dolphins in isolation.

In August 1995 Eve and her mother, Brigitte, were at the Human Dolphin Institute in Panama City Beach. Shizuko, could not go with them because she had to nurse her husband who had been diagnosed with cancer. Instead a Japanese reporter, Saiko Nozaki, who worked for *Amerika Yomiuri*, a Japanese newspaper published in Washington, joined the group to record what happened.

With Brigitte facilitating the use of her hip machine, Eve kept her own journal. I was given a copy of the full record, plus an abbreviated version as an open letter.

20 September 1995

Three weeks ago we were splashing around in the
Gulfstream off the coast of Florida. Was that experience
only a wonder-dappled interlude between waking and
sleeping, or did it mean something well below the
surface of what it appeared to be? Rascals that those
dolphins are, it's quite likely they were playing good
jokes on us and are smiling even wider than usual. At
the time we were actually swimming with them, they
sailed around us checking me out with their clicks. We
could hear them saying to each other 'What do you
make of this weird creature, does she fit the standard
model or is she some new sub species?'

Saiko Nozaki wrote her own account of these events, as an
objective outsider, in an article entitled 'Eve Dreamtime':

Eve Hanf-Enos, a 23-year-old autistic poet and the
president of the Dilo Group, and her mother, Brigitte,
were invited by the Human Dolphin Institute based in
Panama City Beach, Florida to swim with the wild
bottlenose dolphins. Panama City Beach, which is
located near the border of the state of Alabama, is
known for its overly friendly bottlenose dolphins.
Though the locals keep feeding the dolphins to attract
them, which is actually a violation of the Marine
Mammal Protection Act, they did come around the
swimmers like myself without bait. (well, we had Eve
instead!).

On 28 August, Eve encountered dolphins in the wild
for the first time. Eve received keen and lengthy
attention from the dolphins though she was just silently
sitting on the edge of the boat. They were very much
aware of her presence even before she went into the
water. When lifejacket-clad Eve went into the water
with Frederick Chotard helping her, a dolphin came

swimming straight to her. Eve seemed a little frightened to me at the time, but she wrote later that day that she felt safe in the water and that the dolphins really 'knew' her.

When I went into the water with Eve on 31 August, I felt very privileged to witness the 'Eve-dolphin encounter' up close. A dolphin approached her, stayed around on and off for about 30 minutes or so. The dolphin was eagerly checking Eve out with sonar. The dolphin made bubbles underwater a couple of times right in front of Eve. We were told that it is very rare that the dolphins stay around for such a long time. The dolphins really had a 'thing' for her. That evening at the dinner table Eve's mother asked me if one of the dishes was good. I said, 'Uh–huh'. And Eve also said 'Uh–huh' right after it. It sounded as if it came from deep inside her body.

Every reporter I have met who has been in the water with wild dolphins, or has watched others frolicking with them, has been drawn into the event. They just cannot remain totally objective, and invariably end up describing their own feelings. This is what happened to Saiko, except in her case there were two forces pulling on her emotional strings. One was the dolphins. The other was Eve – who by virtue of her abnormality made Saiko question and change her own normality. She described what seeing Eve with the dolphins did to her:

Spending a week with Eve and the dolphins opened a new perspective on communication. Though Eve may be dying to 'speak out' right this minute, words are becoming something of an obsolete way of communication to me. Eve's communication style is very 'open' though some may think that autistic people are handicapped people who must be treated to 'open up' to the outer world and 'speak up'. In Eve's case, her writing puts one of her feet in verbal communication and they may think that Eve is 'opening up' or partially 'cured' or whatever. To me, it seemed as though she is 'speaking' all the time in her own language, but we just don't hear it. She communicates to us by just 'being' herself.

Apart from her writing, Eve's communication style mainly involves sensing, intuiting, and feeling. When I first met Eve in June, I felt as if I fell in a timeless dimension when her eyes captured me. I felt totally exposed. It was as though her eyes were 'reading' my whole existence and there was nowhere to hide. It may not be a coincidence that I felt exactly the same way when I encountered the wild spotted dolphins for the first time. Being utterly exposed. No words, no excuses, and no deceptions. There was no other way but to be 'open' and 'honest'.

If the dolphins communicate or live in 'total honesty' with each other, it might have been a very refreshing experience for them to meet Eve – a human being with 'clear' head. Some scientists claim that dolphins are able to detect each other's emotions by their sonars. If that is true, maybe the dolphins can't help living in total honesty – and maybe felt as though they had spotted one of them when they found Eve.

So what about the dolphins 'healing' Eve? Forget it. Who said autism is an illness anyway? Eve and the dolphins just exist in their 'let me get to your core' kind of human-law defying world. Maybe it's not really Eve who needs to change but we – the 'non-autistic' people – who have really got to change and open up. And who knows? Maybe Eve will someday tell us how to communicate better with the dolphins. When Eve starts speaking, we will be able to share more of her 'dolphin secrets' in person.

Michel Atlas, very wisely, did not raise any expectations of a great improvement in Eve's condition when he undertook to introduce her to the dolphins of Panama City Beach. Upon return to Connecticut Eve wrote of a short period of euphoria which 'was followed by low sagging mood with no appetite for two days'.

Eve's secret desire, to speak using 'lipwords' as she put it, had not been fulfilled. She asked in an open letter to her Dilo friends if any of them could offer an explanation as to why she felt low after experiencing such a high. Her letter ended on a questioning optimistic note:

20 September 1995

Lolling in water, dolphins I hear laughing among themselves, and next time we're in their company I'm sure I'll be laughing with them. Up ahead loom changes in life direction, but I don't feel as frazzled and hassled as in previous changes, so maybe the dolphins know what they're doing. God is disguised as a dolphin, maybe. Jolly sense of humour he has . . . Gone are the gripings about jipped life so I'm quite sure there's a plan behind all this. Millions of dolphins can't be wrong.

Love, Eve

I have always been reluctant to ascribe the beneficial effects of dolphins to some supernatural power, so God disguised as a dolphin I wouldn't accept. But I did accept that there seemed to be some indefinable higher power that was taking us forward in a positive way.

Sadly by 1995, time was running out for Eve's mother. Brigitte had been diagnosed with cancer and her health was deteriorating. It was decided to move Eve, who had been living with her mother and her grandmother in Connecticut, to her own house in New Hampshire where she would be looked after by a new team of 'shadows' as Eve called them. Facilitated writing requires a very special bond between the facilitator and the facilitated. Sometimes it just doesn't work at all. When it does it requires mutual empathy and takes a lot of time and dedication. Also Shizuko, who was looking after her sick husband, could not visit Eve and Brigitte as often as she wished.

Eve lapsed into a period of silence. No more letters arrived after September 1995. Brigitte eventually died in the autumn of 1996. So too did Shizuko's husband, Cornelius (shortened to Kees in Dutch), at the age of 76. Kees was the opposite of Shizuko in many ways. He was tall, handsome, urbane, of good family, and had an air of academic superiority that was close to arrogance. He was interested in facts that could be proved. He was disdainful of the airy-fairy types Shizuko associated with. That is until he met Eve and Brigitte, with whom he had a common bond because they both had cancer. Eve looked Kees in the eyes with her penetrating gaze. She made him realise he was mortal after all and he started to soften. His sense of humour, which most of his life he had kept hidden beneath a stern exterior, started to emerge like sprouting grass. He openly joked with people who previously held him in awe and had remained at a distance. Shizuko told me it was 'a precious experience' to discover this side of her husband's personality. 'Cancer liberated his love', she told me.

When I met Kees, I discovered that we both had a liking for the poetry of Dylan Thomas, and that Kees was an authority on the Welsh poet. Having decided that perhaps I wasn't such a bad chap after all he started to read some of my books.

The playfulness of the dolphins I described somehow rubbed off on him. Kees rediscovered the joys of childhood that he had kept locked away like jewels in a safe. He started playing pranks. One day he visited a local supermarket with Shizuko. He walked out with a large pumpkin on his head which he didn't pay for. Nobody noticed it, or if they did they didn't mention it. When Shizuko told me about the incident we both imagined what would have happened if he had been challenged. We envisaged the scene as being like Monty Python's dead parrot sketch with Kees taking the part of a highly indignant John Cleese.

'Hum, excuse me professor, you have a pumpkin on your head.'

'No I haven't.'

'Yes you have.'

'No I haven't.'

'Yes you have.'

'That is not a pumpkin. That's a hat.'

'No it's not.'

'Yes it is. It's a spherical hat.'

'People don't wear spherical hats.'

'Yes they do.'

'No they don't.'

'Well I do.'

etc.

Shizuko later told me that she couldn't believe the changes that took place in her husband during the last two years of his life.

'Every day he became more like a dolphin,' she told me. Then she amended her statement. 'Well, not so much a dolphin, more an orca.'

'When he knew he had cancer it was like a gift for him,' Shizuko told me. 'I watched him change. He became *so* happy,' she emphasised the word 'so'. 'I would like to make a happiness memorial to him. Kees discovered dolphin happiness in your books and videos. I want others to do so also. I want International Dolphin Watch to set up a Dolphin Happiness Group. I want IDW to give away your books, and any dolphin items that will make people happy. But they should not keep them. They should pass them on, so that dolphin happiness spreads wider and wider.'

It was a typical Shizuko gesture. She gave International Dolphin Watch a cheque to get the scheme under way and said she hoped it would inspire others to do something similar.

After the death of Kees, Shizuko was able to devote more attention to Eve. Shizuko visited Eve in May 1999 and took part, with Eve's grandmother, Lottie (now well into her eighties), her doctor, carers and others, in a discussion group to review Eve's situation. When I read the minutes of the meeting I discovered that Brigitte's habit of leaving no stone unturned was living on. Eve's medication was discussed and arrangements made for Eve to be given a course on a new treatment. It involved Secretin, a drug that has been found to have beneficial effects in others with autism, and works by helping to correct some digestive disorders.

All of the items in the report were positive. Eve was communicating again with a personal computer, on which she composed a short letter to Shizuko and thanked her for giving her so much love. Plans were also proposed for Eve's father to visit her from England. It concluded with the hope that Eve would return to Florida to meet the dolphins again.

I also reviewed Eve's situation privately. It seemed to me that although not using 'lipwords', her world had opened up enormously through her connection to dolphins. Dolphins communicated with her at a deep level which was beyond words. I felt also that Eve had communicated with some humans in a similar way, with a direct transmission of feelings, thoughts and emotions, in which there was no dishonesty.

This caused me to try and put myself in her shoes and ask myself, 'What would the world be like if we could all read one another's thoughts?' If our feelings were totally transparent, the way in which we conduct much of our lives would have to be radically different. In some respects it would be quite frightening.

Another thought crossed my mind. Just as depression can be regarded as a shield behind which a person hides from life's harsh realities, is Eve's autism also a defence mechanism? If so, then dragging her into a world of verbal communication might make us feel better about what we had achieved, but what would it do for Eve? It might possibly do far more harm than good, especially if Eve's autism is an outward manifestation of psychological problems related to deeply disturbing experiences with humans, as is implied in her writings.

Eve's mother, Brigitte, was utterly convinced her daughter could speak if she wanted to. Getting Eve to resolve the problems that caused her to put up the barrier of not speaking

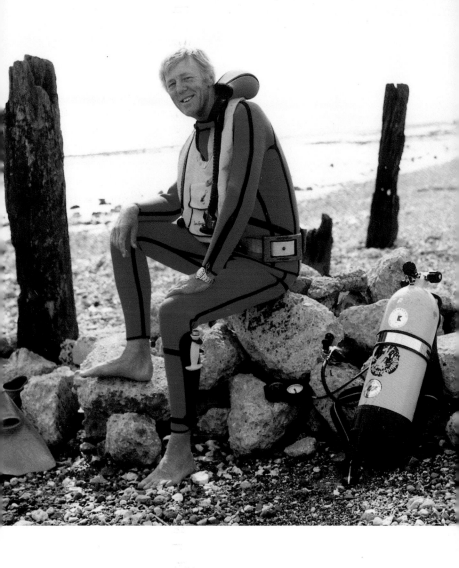

Learning to scuba dive started me on a magical trail of discovery, the outcome of which I never anticipated in my wildest dreams.

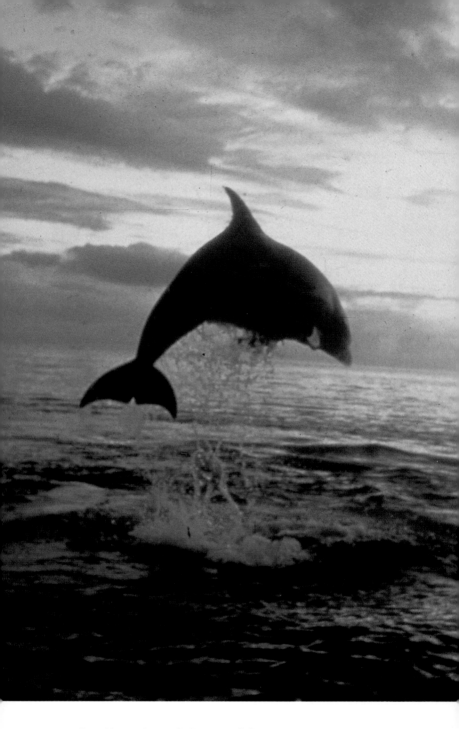

Donald, seen here in high spirits off Cornwall, broke new ground in human/dolphin relationships during his odyssey around Britain in the 1970s.

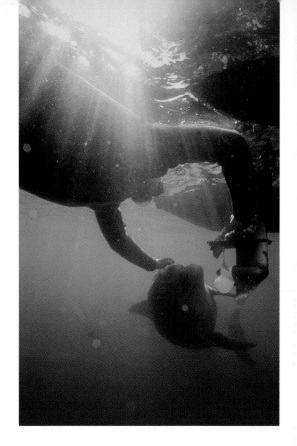

Right: Bill Bowell, who lived in the black hole of chronic depression for many years, saw some light when he met a friendly dolphin in the open sea.

Below: Diver Mike Benison extends the hand of friendship to Fungie, who began to touch human hearts as soon as he arrived in Dingle Bay, Co. Kerry.

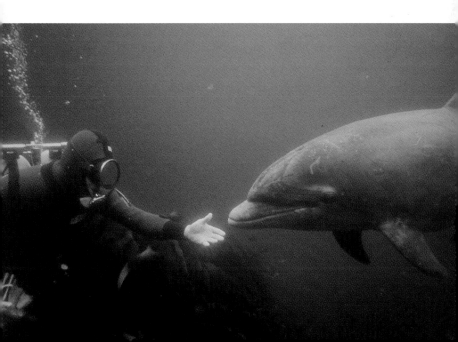

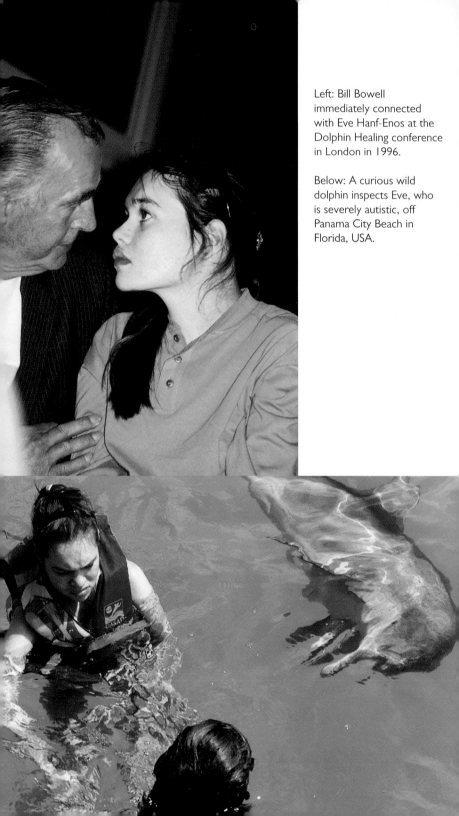

Left: Bill Bowell immediately connected with Eve Hanf-Enos at the Dolphin Healing conference in London in 1996.

Below: A curious wild dolphin inspects Eve, who is severely autistic, off Panama City Beach in Florida, USA.

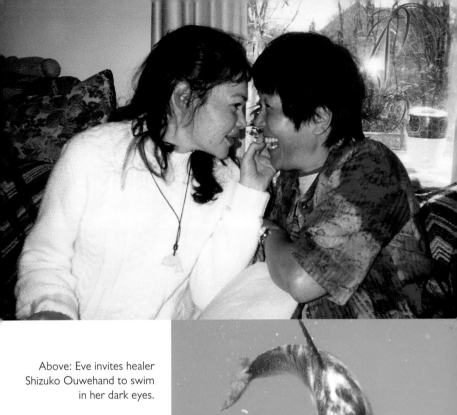

Above: Eve invites healer Shizuko Ouwehand to swim in her dark eyes.

Right: Mike Cowan, an outstanding free diver, being buzzed by a posse of young male spotted dolphins on Rebecca Fitzgerald's Dolphinswim programme in the Bahamas.

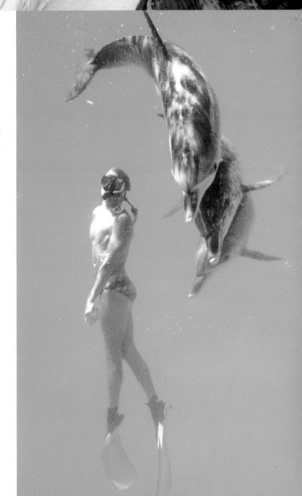

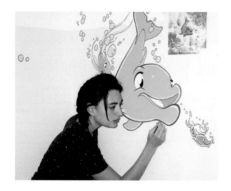

Left: Italian artist Sally Galotti painting Dilo on the wall in a Romanian hospice for children with AIDS.

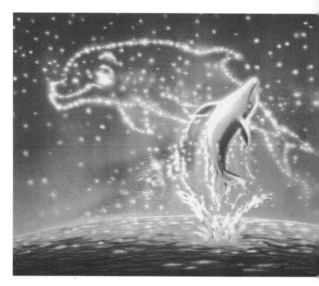

Right: Sally's most popular picture showed Dilo, the mischievous dolphin, jumping for joy when he saw his dead mother in the stars. The children, who had all lost their parents, connected instantly with the painting.

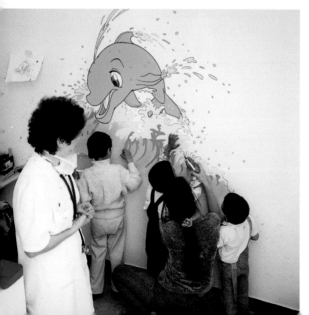

Left: The deep-felt love that Sally expressed in her paintings of Dilo reinforced the joyous survival instincts of many of the children and called into question the prognosis that their AIDS should automatically classify them as terminal patients.

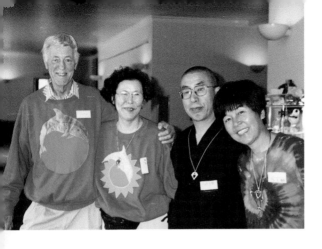

Left: Shizuko (far right) and me (far left) with Konoe and Kokyo Ishizaki who founded the Dolphin Healing Centre in Kyoto.

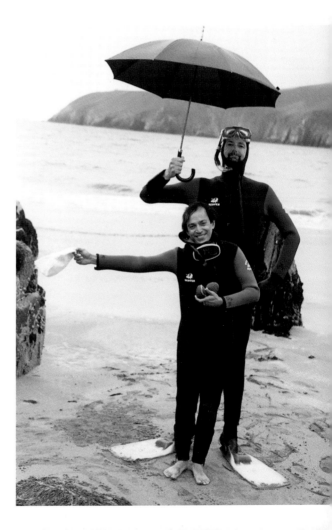

Right: Composer Alec Roth (with umbrella) and librettist Vikram Seth were imbued with a dolphin-like sense of fun when they started work on a new community opera for the ENO in Dingle. Over three hundred youngsters, many with mental and physical disabilities, took part in *Arion and the Dolphin* when it was performed in Plymouth in 1994.

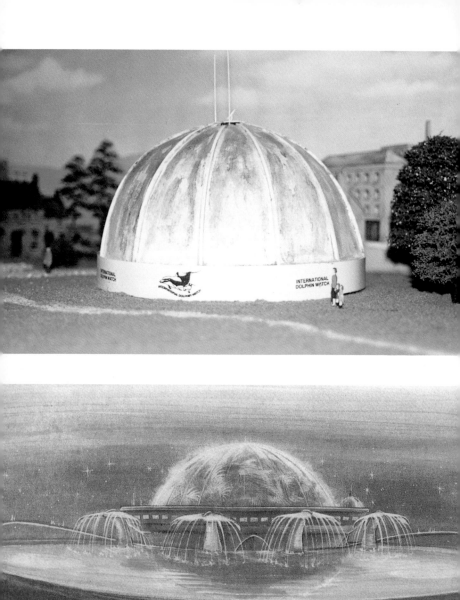

Trevor Goldsmith's first model of a Dilo Dome (top), in which severely disabled children could have interactive sensory dolphin experiences, was followed by a design (illustrated by Sally Galotti, above) for a giant dome in which large audiences could also have amazing experiences, surrounded by waterfalls cascading from full-size whale tails.

is, in my view, fundamentally far more important than cajoling her to say a few more words, although speaking may indicate an improvement in her condition. From the evidence we have so far, I feel strongly that the dolphins, with their apparent total openness, could definitely help Eve in the future. The way forward, therefore, is for Eve to have further encounters with dolphins. If and when this happens, however, it is vitally important that she is with someone who is extremely sensitive to what is going on. She needs to be with a person who will be conscious of the tiniest subtleties of what is happening. When I considered this possibility, the people who came to mind, who might take on this role of interfacing Eve with one or more wild dolphins, were Tricia Kirkman, Bill Bowell, Jemima Biggs or Shizuko Ouwehand. The latter three had all met Eve and each had an empathy with her which went beyond anything I, as a researcher, could proffer. I could, however, act as observer, and afterwards assess what progress, if any, had been made in consultation with those who were closest to her.

When pondering on this future possibility for Eve a thought came into my mind which was a step forward from Rebecca's suggestion of recalling good memories in place of bad ones. Nobody, absolutely nobody, forgets having joyful encounters with dolphins. So how about creating new positive dolphin experiences that will become lasting good memories?

An analogy that supports this logic is the transformation of a refuse tip in North Ferriby on the banks of the River Humber, where I live. In 1980 Riverside Walkway, as it is now called, was a hideous dumping ground, covered with household and industrial waste. In 1982 dumping stopped and it was capped with a thin layer of soil. Now, due in no small degree to the efforts of my wife, Wendy, it is a pleasant, apparently natural recreational area, populated by rabbits and visited by deer and humans. Five thousand trees and shrubs are slowly transforming the underlying trash into glorious life forms that feed flocks of birds and nourish the spirits of the people who stroll amongst them.

The parallel with Eve is that now she has recognised that in the past she had terrible problems, the time has come to bury them, not keep raking them over. She needs to cover them and put something beautiful on top of them. Hopefully, future experiences with the dolphins will, like the wild roses and native trees that now flourish on Riverside Walkway, slowly transform the hidden horrors in her subconscious mind. A sign that this is happening could be that Eve will blossom with 'lipwords'.

Chapter 15
Gala Performance

Dolphin energy was also responsible for inspiring and encouraging a group of disabled children to achieve something which many would have thought impossible – and the inspiration came from Fungie. When the opera *Arion and the Dolphin* (see chapter 3) finally came to fruition it was dedicated by the librettist to Fungie with a poem:

> Irish dolphin, swift and single,
> Dwelling off the coast of Dingle,
> Choosing now and then to mingle
>   With the flipperless and glum,
>
> Bringing wonder and elation
> To our jaded human nation,
> I present you this creation
>   Of my fingers and my thumb.

> [Vikram Seth, from *Arion and the Dolphin, a
> libretto* by Vikram Seth (Phoenix House, 1994)]

I can imagine the amount of work that must go into the production of a well-established opera by a professional company prior to its performance. It must be enormous. The effort required to bring a brand new opera that in addition to using professional performers also involves hundreds of local people, including many disabled children from four schools, plus the conversion of a drill hall into an opera house, I find mind boggling. Yet it happened.

I first met the composer, Alec Roth, in Dingle. He was very tall, slim, conservatively dressed and carried a black rolled umbrella. He was the type who would look completely at home dressed in a pinstripe suit and a bowler hat and would have passed muster on the London Underground as a serious-minded businessman.

When I first saw Alec I mused on how I had become conditioned to relate a person's appearance to his or her role in society. The same situation did not apply with dolphins. Yet they had highly evolved social structures when they were in groups. To me most dolphins looked very similar. Without uniforms or dress codes were they able to tell how they all fitted into their respective slots – if indeed such things existed in their societies? If they did, how did they do it? Do dolphins have auras, or hidden emanations, that other dolphins can recognise and read? I felt instinctively that they had a way of communicating that was beyond anything tangible and measurable to humans.

My mind wandered along this thought line because of something Alec had said to me during our brief introduction. Alec told me that it was not a sight, but the sound of the dolphin that he had first experienced when he arrived in Dingle. He had walked around the bay, following a path along the cliff tops. Everything was still. And then he heard it. A sharp exchange of air – like the release of pressure on the air brakes of a lorry. He looked across the millpond flat sea, but could see no sign of Fungie. Then it happened again as the dolphin snatched another breath before sliding, as silently as a snake, back into the depths of the sea, leaving no other indication of his presence. Thus Alec's first awareness of the presence of Fungie in Dingle Harbour was a sound image – the sound of the dolphin's breath from afar.

It could be argued that Alec's interest in the dolphin breathing was an integral part of his work as a composer. Breathing is vitally important for opera singers. For an aria to work properly the breaths, the words and the music have to fit together with the precision of a watch mechanism. Despite this I felt there was much more to Alec's first awareness of Fungie than a simple response to the sound of the dolphin breathing. A bond, more spiritual than physical, had been formed between them before he had even seen Fungie.

Alec and I, and the rest of the English National Opera team, all stayed at the same bed and breakfast run by Peggy O'Connor. It was situated in a farmhouse on the western outskirts of Dingle. Stunning views of Dingle Bay, and the distant misty mountains of the Macgillycuddy Reeks, that rose to over 3400 metres, were visible from the upstairs bedrooms. With binoculars it was sometimes possible to spot Fungie fishing, especially when he tossed a prize salmon in the air.

To the west lay Slea Head and the notorious Blasket Islands where many seafarers had come to grief. It was to this most western tip of Europe that the team from ENO mustered for the very first run through of the libretto.

For me Slea Head is one of the most spectacular and dramatic seascapes on earth. We stopped off on the way to inspect some beehive houses built by the earliest known inhabitants of the peninsula over a thousand years earlier. These extraordinary dwellings were made from stones piled together in the form of domes. The tangible sense of history and mystery that pervaded them prepared us for the step back in time we were about to make when we immersed ourselves in the story of Arion which is centred around Periander, the tyrannical King of Corinth in about 600 BC. Like many megalomaniacs, Periander was a patron of the arts. Arion, who was reputed to be the best harp player of his day, was one of those who found favour with the king.

After spending some time in the Royal Court, Arion travelled to the Greek colonies in Italy and Sicily. Arion won the contests for musicians and poets that were run alongside athletic competitions in Sicily. He amassed a fortune before triumphantly setting off on his return journey to Corinth. En route Arion fell foul of the greed and envy of the crew of the ship that was carrying the fêted musician and his treasures. They plotted to kill him. But it was hard to keep the secret on a small vessel. When Arion got to hear of their plans, he begged for his life. They refused.

'Then let me sing to you one last time before I die,' he pleaded.

Arion's wish was granted. The musician/poet dressed in his finery, played his lyre and sang more beautifully than ever. Dolphins, attracted to the sound, escorted the vessel as it sailed on. The crew were mesmerised by Arion's performance. They watched dumbfounded when the singer suddenly jumped overboard to join the dolphins.

One of the dolphins carried Arion ashore, and the rescued musician made his way back to Periander's court in Corinth, minus his treasure. The king suspected some nefarious plan to defraud him of his share of the wealth. He didn't believe the poet's improbable account of being condemned to death and then rescued by the dolphins. So Arion was imprisoned.

When the sailors returned they told Periander they had taken Arion back to his home on the Island of Lesbos. Arion's presence in prison in Corinth contradicted their story. He was set free and completely exonerated. Arion's fame was greater than ever.

As a tribute to the gods for his rescue Arion placed an offering, in the form of a small bronze figure of a man riding on a dolphin, in the temple at Tainaron where he was brought ashore. The historian Herodotus saw the statuette 200 years later. It convinced him of the authenticity of the account of Arion's rescue which he had heard, and had been passed down from mouth to mouth by the people of Corinth.

A story like that of Arion and the dolphins must have an exceptionally magical quality for its appeal to endure. Had Herodotus returned over 24 centuries later, I wonder what he would have thought of the latest version being told by the theatrical troupe on a headland in Ireland? I am sure he would have approved of the magnificent setting for the performance.

Our stage was a bed of spongy grass festooned with orchids, wort, vetch, trefoil and a host of other wild flowers overlooking Dunquin. Far below us on a small landing were the black upturned hulls of a dozen or so currachs. The origin of these lightweight rowing boats is hidden in the mists of time. Similar vessels, consisting of canvas stretched over a light wooden lattice frame, were almost certainly used to ferry the earliest settlers to and from the Blasket Islands. From our platform high on the cliffs we could clearly see the once populated outcrops. Between us lay a deceptively peaceful-looking, sparkling sea, its treacherous currents and submerged rocks lying in wait to claim any inexperienced, or unlucky sailors. Beyond the islands, the Atlantic Ocean stretched unbroken to North America.

Vikram Seth distributed copies of his first attempt at the libretto. We were each given different roles to speak.

The opera opens in the Court of King Periander (Alec Roth), where Arion, played by Vikram Seth, is pleading to be released to sing in Sicily. The heading in Scene 2 reads: *As Arion sings to the sea, the CAPTAIN and the SAILORS appear and begin to sing; and the scene changes to shipboard as the trumpet Theme of Corinth grows fainter.*

'We have no musical instruments,' said Vikram, 'but Horace has his magnificent didgeridoo. 'Horace,' He paused and theatrically raised one arm to the heavens. 'Horace' he announced, 'shall be our orchestra.' Another pause, 'The sound of trumpets please maestro!'

I made tooting sounds on my didgeridoo. 'Wonderful, wonderful!,' exclaimed Vikram with enthusiasm, 'Let us continue'.

The Dutch stage designer Henk Schut took the role of the ship's captain whose emotions are torn between greed for Arion's treasure and compassion for the life of the musician. Rebecca Meitlis, founder and producer of the project, spoke various minor parts as did Angie, one of whose jobs back in London is that of production manager.

And so the tale of *Arion and the Dolphin* unfolds, with Vikram using liberal amounts of artistic licence in his interpretation of the classic tale. He also brings the story into the twentieth century with the capture, and death in captivity, of the dolphin who rescued our eponymous hero.

I was surprised and pleased at this twist in the plot. The captivity issue was one for which I have campaigned ever since I first met Donald, who forcefully made me realise that all dolphins have the right to swim free in the sea.

These happenings on the cliff tops made me ponder, yet again, on what strange forces were moving humanity. How could a single, selfless act by a dolphin change the lives of thousands of people? How 2600 years later, could that same dolphin, through music, bring joy and thereby healing into the lives of disadvantaged children? For that is precisely what happened when the opera was eventually performed. *Arion and the Dolphin* had its first gala performance on Friday 17 June 1994 and I was there with my wife Wendy to witness it, and be part of it.

It was an immensely pleasurable event. A thinly veiled, lemon-yellow sun, still high in the sky, transformed what could have been a bleak windswept hillside into a fairytale setting. It illuminated the scene below with soft light, giving the people and the buildings an ethereal quality. It could have been a film set. A frisson of anticipation filled the air. This was not just another night at the opera for a gathering of seasoned, well-heeled toffs. No, this was a night for a great gathering of ordinary folk. Many of them, parents of mentally and physically disabled children, had never been to an opera before. And they were here because their little Johnny, or their little Mary, was actually taking part.

This was what *Arion and the Dolphin* was all about. It was a community opera. It was part of the Baylis Programme of the ENO, the intention of which was to widen the appeal of opera, and encourage everyone and anyone to participate, and enjoy it. Alec Roth had worked for months beforehand, encouraging and tutoring over 300 youngsters, many with mental and physical disabilities, to sing and play music. Tonight was their big night.

If you wanted to find any place in the world less imposing, or conducive to the sensitivity of a great musical occasion, you would find it hard to beat the drill hall at HMS Drake, the present name for the Royal Navy barracks at Devonport. The building itself is as basic as it gets.

Those responsible for putting on the opera had a very limited budget derived mainly from sponsors. To convert a drill shed into a temporary opera house was out of the question. Scaffolding was the primary material for the construction of the stage. Sheets of plastic draped from the ceiling were cleverly used to create above water and underwater scenes. In other words it was not the kind of situation where the audience was instantly transported into a make-believe world by glamorous surroundings and an elaborate stage set, which is part and parcel of going to see a live show – especially opera. The magic that would lift the audience into a realm of fantasy would have to come entirely from the players.

And it did.

My lack of practical knowledge of music meant that I was blissfully unaware of any technical hitches. I just absorbed it as a whole, and thoroughly enjoyed it. The scenes in which lots of youngsters took part, dancing across the stage between sheets of blue plastic, to become dolphins under the sea, I found enchanting. When they accidentally bumped into one another it added to the joyful, carefree, playground atmosphere the children were trying to convey.

At the end of the performance the audience loudly clapped its approval and appreciation. When the applause faded proud parents and grandparents hurried into the crowded, makeshift dressing rooms to gather up their excited chattering offspring and their outfits. They then made their way to the lawns for the finale – a spectacular firework display. The grand gala performance of *Arion and the Dolphin* was formally brought to a close by a solitary bugler playing The Last Post.

When we eventually left HMS Drake there was still some light in the sky. It was close to the summer solstice. As we made our way back to the car park I pondered yet again on the extraordinary chain of events that had led me to Plymouth, and how unbelievably filled with joy my life had become since I met Donald the dolphin, almost exactly 20 years earlier. I also knew that the magic would not stop here. Our hosts at the bed and breakfast, to which we were heading, had their own role to play in my ongoing magical journey into dolphin healing.

Music had already played a key role in the form of Dolphin Dreamtime. At the Ki and Dolphin Healing Centre in Kyoto music took on yet another cloak. Shortly before our arrival for the opening Konoe, the wife of the priest, was inspired to write a melody which has that very special quality that makes it stick in your mind and keep repeating itself. Japanese words were added. When the proceedings were under way, Shizuko, who has a beautiful voice, sang it and then got everyone to sing along. It was titled *Iruka No Uta* – the Song of the The Dolphin, or The Dolphin Song (see page 178).

A Japanese musician, the owner of a much prized American trumpet made in the 1930s, gave a virtuoso performance of the dolphin melody in a variety of styles, from blues to rock and roll.

When the German musician Radha first heard the melody, she thought it was a traditional Japanese song. She didn't know where it originated and made an entire CD based upon the Iruka theme.

I have an immense love of music, but I cannot play a musical instrument – unless you count the didgeridoo! When I hear the piano recording of Iruka by Radha, it touches me in subconscious ways that strangely liberate my mind. Although I have never measured them, I am sure it changes my electrical brain-wave patterns. I find listening to Radha's version of Iruka ideal when taking a short instant sleep, which I do often. I also play it on repeat on my CD player when I am engaged in the protracted process of creative writing. My books are very personal and to me they are alive. When I write I feel as if I am speaking directly to whoever eventually reads them. For some totally idiosyncratic reason I have found by long experience that the best route for my words to find emergence into printed form is via longhand scribble on the backs of used sheets of paper on a clipboard.

As my mind has a tendency to go into butterfly mode when I am writing, my longhand often gets into the most tangled state, with many transportations of words and phrases. It was therefore with some embarrassment that I presented the chapters of the manuscript for this book to Susie, at nearby Redcliff Studios to be transformed, nay transmogrified, into the text you are now reading. In defence of this preposterous procedure I venture to reiterate one of the precious lessons that Cheryl Hutchins and the dolphins have taught me. It is be who I am, not what others may expect me to be.

Chapter 16
Dolphin Domes

Shortly before setting off to attend the gala performance of *Arion and the Dolphin* in Plymouth, I found a note on my desk from the Education Officer of International Dolphin Watch.

> Leila Edwards wrote to me recently asking for info re dolphins into schools project. She offers accommodation if required during your stay in Plymouth for the opera gala. Leila is Director of Student Services and Acting Assistant Principal at Plymouth College of Further Education.

The note included an address and telephone number. I accepted Leila's kind offer of accommodation and liked her and her house immediately we stepped inside the door. We soon got into animated conversation. As my wife and Leila engaged in noisy chatter I became involved in deep discussion with Leila's husband Phil, who I discovered was doing research on sensory environments.

Phil explained how, using equipment available relatively cheaply from theatrical suppliers, he could create a whole range of completely different environments from quiet to noisy, from dark to light, and from static to mobile. Furthermore these were interactive. The different elements could be controlled by breaking ultrasound beams, of the type used in some burglar alarms. Interrupting the beams in different places could trigger a range of effects that were widely variable. Swiping a finger through the beam at one point could set off a recording of a symphony orchestra. Cutting the beam at other points could activate a recording of waves lapping the shore, or rock and roll music.

Phil showed me a video he had made demonstrating his experimental assembly in action. He explained how he wished to carry out further research to a standard that would lead to his qualifying for a higher degree. Phil's combination of art and science had obvious applications to what I was trying to do in my attempts to recreate artificially an interaction with a dolphin. Using variations of Phil's rig I could generate a whole gamut of different sensations which could convey the excitement and joy of meeting a dolphin, especially with a wide range of visual and sound effects.

I had already conceived the idea of a dolphin therapy pool, in which the participant would become part of a healing aquatic environment. But this concept had limitations, not the least of which was the expense of construction and maintenance of a pool. The idea of creating a range of different sensory stimulations by adapting low cost and readily available equipment was immensely exciting. It opened up a whole new territory for dolphin healing which could make it universally available. Before that could happen, however, a lot of research would have to be done.

When we left Plymouth I had a clear idea in my mind about how we should set about this. My long-term aim was to create an interactive sensory unit, incorporating different elements of dolphin healing. It could be static or mobile. I had no doubts in my mind that a suitable project could be devised that would contain sufficient novel research to make it acceptable by a university as a thesis for a PhD. However, there was one major obstacle to taking the proposal forward. Money. Phil would have to obtain research grants. As a father with teenage children he had responsibilities. His needs were not excessive, but reverting to the life of an impecunious student for three years or more was not an option. International Dolphin Watch had extremely limited funds and couldn't help.

Time went by. Phil and I continued to develop our ideas on the role interactive sensory environments might play in dolphin healing. An application to the National Lottery was turned down. As we later rattled our brains to find a way to resolve this problem, Phil's personal circumstances changed. His wife Leila got a new job and they moved from Plymouth. A short time later the project had a fresh impetus. A new player, Trevor Goldsmith, came into the game.

Trevor was an extraordinarily creative man who I first met at one of my playshops at Flint House in Lewes, East Sussex. He was a commercial fisherman and had his own small fishing boat based in nearby Newhaven. At the playshop he revealed that he liked to listen to Mozart when he was fishing. He often had dolphins around his boat. His dream was to design a boat to introduce underprivileged children to the ways of the sea, especially dolphins. This ambition was completely compatible with my aims for International Dolphin Watch. It provided the common ground upon which we soon built a powerful friendship.

Trevor Goldsmith came to visit me at my home shortly after I met him at Flint House. It was then that I discovered more about the modest fisherman with his own dream. The man was a genius. He was a superb sculptor, a brilliant boat designer and a remarkable marine-life researcher. In addition he had very strong moral principles concerning the manner in which the products of his fertile mind should be carried forward to realise their commercial potential. In this respect I realised, from personal experience with ruthless businessmen, that Trevor had a certain commercial naiveté that he himself recognised, and that had cost him dear. But for me that was part of what I found attractive about him. He also had an uncontrollable enthusiasm for developing new ideas that continuously stretched his personal financial resources to the limit.

One of the things that brought us closer together was a new idea I had. How about putting an interactive sensory environment inside a dome? This concept came to me after a presentation made by the musician and storyteller Ken Shapley at The Dolphin Healing Conference in London in June 1996 where he set out to recreate the essence of dolphins and confine it within a healing space. This he created by draping translucent blue fabric over a prototype dome-shaped frame, rather like a tent. Light from outside illuminated the interior with a blue glow. Images of dolphins painted on the fabric gave those lying face-up inside the feeling that they were under the sea, surrounded by dolphins. The magic was completed when Ken filled the inside of his dome with the haunting music of his didgeridoo.

Phil Edwards' experiments had been conducted in a large industrial unit in which the equipment needed to produce the various effects was there for all to see. In the dolphin healing dome I imagined, none of this would be on show. Only the effects the various gadgets produced would be apparent. I did not want those inside the dome to be distracted by machines. My plan was for those going into the dome to feel that they were entering a space in which magical events could take place. It was to be a place in which they could play with sound and visual images. Just moving a finger in and out of the beams would activate a plethora of different sensory experiences. The inside of the dome would be the ultimate playground, in which the adult, or child, could shed all of their problems and become lost in a dolphin fantasy.

In March 1997 I put forward this concept to members of International Dolphin Watch in the form of a proposal, The Dolphin Dome Project. In the article I explained how art, science and technology overlapped in the creation of an artificial dolphin experience that could be researched to develop therapy programmes, especially for the severely disabled.

Shortly afterwards I announced plans to move the entire concept another step forward, to a what I dubbed the Double Dome. This consisted of two domes, one inside the other. The space in between them was where the machinery needed to operate the various effects would be accommodated and hidden from view, rather like a hemispherical mezzanine floor in a building. Thus from the outside it would look like a simple dome, and entering it would also be like going into a simple single dome. Inside the sonic, visual and tactile aspects of the dolphin images could be varied by the patients. The machines could also be overidden and controlled by the operators. Thus we could investigate and evaluate which aspects of our simulated dolphin experiences were most beneficial to those with autism and other neurological dysfunctions.

In October 1997 provisional plans were drawn up to construct a Double Dolphin Dome that could be dismantled and transported in a pantechnicon. This had been made possible by Trevor who applied his boat-building skills to the design of ribs that could be assembled into dome shapes, and dismantled quickly for easy transport. The pantechnicon would enable us to take the dome to different centres where it could be evaluated by specialists working with patients with special needs.

The logical way forward for such a project was to do the research first and then, from that, derive therapy programmes. Both Trevor and I were far too impatient to go through this long-winded process which would take years and be very difficult to finance. We knew that our proposed dome had numerous conventional commercial applications, even if we did not know the optimal working conditions for therapy. So we decided to go for a dome that could be used straightaway, and to operate it out-of-hours for structured scientific studies.

Everyone with whom I discussed the Mobile Double Dolphin Dome Project thought it was a wonderful idea. Surprisingly, it turned out to be a fictional dolphin, Dilo, and an Italian artist, Sally Galotti, who were to play a role in taking the project another step forward.

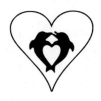

Chapter 17
The Dilo Dome

It was the response of the audience to *Arion and the Dolphin* that brought home to me, once again, the powerful emotions that could be evoked by dolphin images of all kinds. The act of taking part had obviously been of therapeutic benefit to the disabled children involved in the actual opera. But it was anybody's guess what part, if any, the fact that a dolphin was involved played in this healing process.

The behaviour of the young woman who became locked on to my picture of Percy the dolphin during my first meeting with Dr Nakagawa (see p. 56) introduced me to the concept that dolphin images could carry their own healing energy. In that case, however, it was an image of a dolphin, Percy, who I knew had his own therapeutic power, that attracted her. But could those seeking help benefit from images of a totally fictional dolphin, a cartoon dolphin, I asked myself?

I had created just such a dolphin and named him Dilo. Although Dilo was a made-up name, all of his antics which I had described in several children's books, were based upon personal experiences. So to me at least, Dilo was a real-life dolphin.

The possibility that Dilo could indeed have a healing role became apparent to me when a young Italian artist, Sally Galotti, stepped into my life. Sally contacted me after she had read the Italian edition of *Journey into Dolphin Dreamtime* in 1996. I knew from her letter that she worked for the Walt Disney organisation and I was delighted when she said she would like to illustrate Dilo in glorious colour. Within a short time Sally found a publisher, Edizione punto d'incontro, who agreed to publish an Italian edition of one of my Dilo books in full colour.

As the weeks passed I discovered Sally possessed a powerful resolution, which, once committed to a project, saw it through, even if it entailed intense and prolonged effort. For nine months Sally worked at the studio in her home in Milan. Occasional sketches came my way. But it was not until the job was complete, and I saw her finished illustrations, that I realised just how much effort she had put into them.

The influence of her background at Disney was apparent in both the style and the content of Sally's brightly coloured images of Dilo. But they were not just commercial Mickey Mouse-like images. There was a captivating humour in them. Even more than that, there was a power in them that came from her soul.

Gradually I became aware of the force that had driven Sally to make such an enormous effort. She wanted to help herself by helping children, especially those infected with AIDS and incarcerated in hospices in Romania. Her inspiration to become involved in this heart-rending cause was the Italian television presenter Mino Damato, who was dedicated to human rights and worked tirelessly to help children. He raised funds, and went to Romania to see that the money was used properly.

Mino accepted an offer of help from Sally. She contributed her talents as an artist. Sally sent me photographs taken on her visits to a hospice where she painted images of Dilo on the walls.

Sally was astounded and overwhelmed by the spirit of the children. They clamoured around her, hugging her and kissing her. What they wanted and needed more than anything else was love. This Sally gave them. She also poured her love into pictures of Dilo which they helped her paint on the walls. A love that would continue to be felt by them when she left.

When we spoke on the phone she told me heartrending stories. One girl, who was 15, but looked more like nine, moved Sally immensely. She sent me a picture of the girl, dressed in pink, helping her to decorate a wall. The little girl died during Sally's next visit. But Sally showed no outward signs of the distress she felt inside when she was at the hospice. Her role was to bring love and joy, not sorrow, into the lives of those who were still alive.

In the final chapter of *Dilo and the Call of the Deep* which was published in Italy, with Sally's illustrations, under the title *Dilo e it richiamo degli abissi*, the young dolphin loses his mother, who dies caught in a net. When Dilo looks up into the sky at night, and sees the dolphin constellation, he recognises his mother outlined in the stars. At that moment the dolphin realises that although his mother is dead, her spirit will always be with him, to guide him and comfort him.

The poignant picture Sally painted of this moment of realisation in Dilo's life was by far the most appreciated in Romania. When she told me this I realised that Dilo was helping the children, and those who cared for them, come to terms with death.

But then Sally mentioned something that took me aback. She said that some of the children had so much spirit she felt they might not die.

I found Sally's suggestion, that some of the children would survive, very compelling. It made me think back to Dr Nakagawa. I had seen him at work. I had been given a book by one of his patients, herself a qualified dentist, in which she revealed how she had been cured of terminal cancer. Shizuko's friend Lilo had made a similar recovery from cancer. Why should I, or anyone else for that matter, just accept the fact that the children with AIDS in Romania were all terminal? Could some of them move off death row with the help of the energy field, which Dr Nakagawa channelled to his patients, and which he claimed was also radiated by live dolphins and dolphin images?

I felt instinctively that the positive attitude Sally adopted towards the situation in Romania could, in combination with other factors, lead to the remission of AIDS in some of the children.

Another significant event which reinforced my thoughts on the healing power of dolphin images occurred in 1998 when Sally and I visited Muller Children's Hospital in Los Angeles. There we met the Executive Director, Dr Mel Marks. His declared aim was to provide the best possible medical care for children in a non-threatening environment.

I gave a presentation on dolphin healing to the staff and some of the patients, explaining my vision for the future, which included an interactive sensory environment inside a Dilo Dome (as the Dolphin Dome came to be known to avoid people thinking it contained a live dolphin show). Dr Marks took us on an extensive tour of the hospital. The corridors were painted with scenes of pirate ships and treasure islands. There were play facilities in the large reception area.

Dr Marks took us into a room where children had their plaster casts removed. 'Look at this,' he said. The room was filled with medical equipment. 'It's daunting to the parents and frightening for the children. Bringing them straight into this kind of environment can be terrifying. So I want to make hospital a fun place to come into. I want children to want to come into my hospital. Happiness is one of the best medicines. Children respond to treatment better, regardless of what is wrong with them, if they are not stressed.'

It was what I wanted to hear. Here was a physician whose aim was to create a joyful, healing environment in his hospital.

Dr Marks could not have been more encouraging and helpful. If we could raise the money, Dr Marks said he would be pleased to have a Dilo Dome in the courtyard. This I realised would provide a valuable opportunity to do research and therapy simultaneously.

Inside the dome I wanted my fictional dolphin, Dilo, to take children into a magical world under the sea. But much more important than that was my wish to use Dilo to help children, especially those who were severely ill, to escape, not just into make-believe fantasy, but into a reality where real improvements in their health were possible.

My visit to California in 1998 was a great learning experience. Upon my return I had an even clearer vision of how Dilo could help children who were ill. I identified the process in a broadsheet I produced for International Dolphin Watch. The front page was a new colourful picture of Dilo by Sally bearing the message:

DILO THE DOLPHIN

brings

Joy, Love and Healing
to the children of the world.

One of those who shared my enthusiasm for the Dilo Dome Project was Ed Bentham at Huron University in Kensington, London. Some of those attending this educational establishment were drawn from families connected with diplomacy, banking and big business. Many came from different parts of the world. As part of their curriculum they were expected to participate in experiential learning programmes. Ed decided that devising a business plan and spread sheet for the construction and running of a dome would be a valuable exercise for his students. He therefore called a meeting at the university at which Trevor and I, plus about 18 others who had been drawn into the Dilo Dome concept were invited to discuss how it should be taken forward.

Several major factors emerged from the debate. The primary one was that domes had virtually unlimited commercial potential. We all agreed that the best way to progress the project was to develop it as a viable commercial venture, not necessarily connected directly with dolphins, but which would provide the facilities and funding for the original objectives to be achieved.

The unique construction principles devised by Trevor allowed for the building of dome-shaped structures of all sizes, from small to gigantic. Thus domes could be developed for different purposes, which ranged from mobile education and exhibition features, to permanent places of entertainment.

According to their size, the various domes could accommodate a variety of internal features, including a waterfall fed by a pool, into which laser images could be projected. This would also be used as a dolphin therapy pool. The latest technological devices used in concerts would be deployed to create an astounding array of sound and visual effects surrounding the pool. Moving pictures could be projected onto giant mist screens. Most of these features would be designed to be interactive, enabling those inside the domes to be involved in creating the overall experience.

To expand his vision Trevor took inspiration from Delphi on Mount Parnassus, the holiest place in Ancient Greece. People came from far and wide to ask their fortunes at the Delphic oracle, to make contact with their gods in the Temple of Apollo, and gather for entertainment in the huge stadium. The town flourished commercially. Through pilgrims' fees and their offerings, Delphi accrued the richest collection of treasures in the Greek world. With this information in the back of his mind, Trevor took the dome concept to the limit. He envisioned a colossal dome surrounded by waterfalls, pouring over huge sculptures of whale tails, into a kind of moat.

On entering the dome visitors would find themselves in a wide circular walkway, depicting sacred architectural themes set in different environments. The plant and animal life beneath the waterfalls could be viewed through windows. Leading off the walkway would be rooms used for a variety of complementary treatments such as aromatherapy. Wheelchair access, available throughout, would lead into the centre of the dome which would have a seating capacity of over 1000 and from which the spectacle in the central arena could be viewed and interacted with.

Trevor told Sally of his vision for this grand dome. She interpreted his sketches and added her own imagination to produce an artist's impression of what the dome would look like, inside and out. Her painting of the dome, set beneath a star-studded sky, was not unlike that of a giant spaceship.

At a gathering at Huron University on 23 November 1999 Trevor was able to announce some exciting news. A major international construction company had made a commitment to the Dilo Dome project. A site for the first prototype dome was being prepared in Ireland. We were on our way.

The structural designs for a mobile dome were also well advanced. So I floated the idea of having a mobile dome tour through Europe to Romania. Several people immediately offered to help raise funds. With this kind and generous support I felt the odds of another dream becoming a reality were good.

Chapter 18
'Eye Search'

ICERC stands for International Cetacean Education Research Centre, which is too much of a mouthful for most people to say. The organisation is almost invariably referred to by its acronym, which conveniently comes out as 'Eye Search' in English.

ICERC was founded by Kamala Hope Campbell, an Australian whose life was changed in 1982 by dolphins who came to her in a dream. Until then, she thought dolphins were fish. In the week that followed she discovered that dolphins were mammals and conscious breathers – awake 24 hours a day. For Kamala, however, the most remarkable characteristic of the dolphins was that they reached out to us humans, no matter what we did to harm them and their large cousins, the whales, who we had hunted nearly to extinction.

In her homeland, Australia, a new consciousness towards dolphins was awakening. The February 1986 issue of the International Dolphin Watch magazine *Dolphin* carried the following letter by one of Kamala's friends.

Dear Dolphin Watchers

The Dolphin Encounter Network has been established to help bridge the gap between man and cetaceans. At present we are giving workshops in Australia using a form of mediation called Dolphin Dreaming.

Using specially designed music and techniques it is possible to open our hearts and minds to the world of cetacea. The Australian aboriginals have been tuning into the Dolphin Dreamworld for thousands of years. It seems that at this time when mankind stands at the crossroads of history, the dolphins and whales are reaching out to make contact and communicate.

During the actual Dolphin Dreaming participants receive messages of hope and often report sensations of physical healing.

The dolphins and whales give so much without hope of reward. Many reports have been documented of dolphins and whales helping humans in time of distress.

There is so much to learn from these wonderful creatures. For me, personally, I have been shown a way to find peace, love and hope.

Happy Dolphin Dreams,

Tara

At the time we published Tara's letter I was completely unaware of the important role Dolphin Dreamtime would eventually play in my explorations of the healing power of dolphins.

A subsequent issue of the magazine announced a forthcoming event in Australia. It was the direct result of Kamala having another dream in 1987, which was to bring together mystics, artists, scientists, conservationists and activists to share their knowledge. The outcome was the first Dolphin and Whale Conference held at Nambucca Heads, New South Wales in May 1988. The global 'Eye Search' family was born.

Another part of Kamala's dream was to set up a centre where people could come together to share their experiences and dreams with others. A site was purchased at Valla Beach. It was Kamala's 'Snowman'. And like my snowman, it didn't work out quite the way it was originally planned. It was superseded by a vision that was even better.

In 1989 a right whale and her baby spent three weeks close to Kamala's home. This led her to have a beautiful and complex vision about Japan. It was that the Japanese people would lead the world into a better understanding of dolphins and whales. As a result a second conference was held at Nambucca Heads in 1990, at which a presentation was given by a brave and active Japanese conservationist, Eiji Fujiwara.

The 20 delegates from Japan who attended the third ICERC Conference in Hawaii in 1992 received a standing ovation. One of those who made a commitment to dolphin conservation was Takako Iwatani. She raised 60 dedicated volunteers to help put together the fourth ICERC Conference which took place in Japan in 1994.

The fifth conference was held in Brussels in 1996. In 1997 Kamala took the conference back to Australia where the focus was on the importance of the connection of indigenous people to the whales and dolphins and on creating a future for the next seven generations. It was opened by an Aboriginal Elder. Auntie Pearl King, whose immensely moving and powerful address brilliantly summed up the situation of the Aborigines, and how she saw the way they must move forward in harmony with the 'white fellas' as she referred to them, who had wrought enormous changes, not all bad, to her homeland.

Shizuko and I attended the seventh ICERC Conference in Japan where Kamala finished her introductory speech as follows:

ICERC is now ten years old and it has grown to be something quite beautiful. Looking at Earth from the moon it is Planet Water and the intelligent beings on it are the dolphins and whales – not us. We have an awesome opportunity to communicate with another species who have so much to teach us about living. We must relate from a place of equality and respect. When communication between the species beyond language happens, Gaia will have made her next evolutionary step.

And so, on Saturday 28 March 1998, the seventh ICERC Conference got under way.

The host of the conference, Takako Iwatani, was a remarkable young woman whose beauty and charm camouflaged a tough interior. Shortly after she undertook to organise the conference, she became pregnant. But she did not let this stop her from fulfilling her obligations. At the height of this awesome task, which involved looking after 400 foreign delegates, she gave birth to a beautiful bouncy boy named Shinki. At just a few weeks old, Shinki was the youngest attendee at the conference.

The event was a glorious party to which many of my dolphin friends including Dr John Lilly, Jim Nollman and Jaques Mayol were invited. There were some compelling new presenters too, including the science journalist Peter Russell.

Dr Bernd Wursig, Director of the Texas A&M University Marine Mammal Research Programme, gave an excellent illustrated talk in which he brilliantly balanced his ecological studies with the emotional attachment he and other scientists felt for the animals they were studying.

The conference also reflected the realisation of Kamala's dream – namely that Japan would play a key role in building a new and harmonious relationship between humans and dolphins. Marike Ukiyo, a well-known Japanese writer and psychological counsellor at the International Mental State Education Centre Corporation, revealed how, through their art, the changes that took place in emotionally disturbed children after contact with dolphins found expression in their paintings, which became happy and full of rainbow colours. Dr Akimitsu Yokoyama, a psychiatrist, spoke about his studies with animal therapy in the Kyosai-Tachikawa Hospital.

Dr Kathleen Durdzinski, a post doctoral fellow from Texas

A&M University, sponsored by the Japanese Society for the Promotion of Science, reported on how she had extended her studies of dolphins in Florida and the Bahamas to the Japanese island of Mikurajima where systematic observations had been gathered by Japanese members of ICERC since 1994. Using a mobile video/acoustic system Kathleen recorded both human and dolphin behaviour in a scientific study of the dolphins themselves, and the effect being joined by swimming humans was having on them. Kathleen's study concentrated on the dolphins, but it was obvious from what she said that the humans were affected too. More seeds of change were being sown which would profoundly change Japanese attitudes to dolphins. After outlining a programme code of conduct for dolphinswim programmes, Kathleen concluded her illustrated presentation:

> It is important to realise that the ocean is not our home, but our playground. It is, however, home to dolphins, whales and other marine organisms. We are guests and should act accordingly.

An additional conference event at Ikoi-no-sato in Mihami-Izu was billed as a 'workshop'. But it should have been called a 'playshop', because that is exactly what it was. Everyone joined in the group activities with collective fun and enthusiasm as only the Japanese can. Most of the participants were young city dwellers, who, when given a taste of what it is like to have contact with nature, became full of dolphin spirit and energy.

In the playshops they were able to step outside the concrete confines of urban life and form joyous relationships with one another. In doing so they were better able to understand the play-filled, group-centred world of the dolphins, which is not governed by competitive commerce and has no boundaries. The changes in their deportment and behaviour before and after showed that all of the youngsters attending the playshops benefited from them. To me this was an example of the role dolphins can have as models towards helping to resolve the emotional problems that can arise from isolation in inner cities – especially amongst the young.

Kamala's dream that the Japanese would lead the way to a new future was further advanced by a series of whale- and dolphin-watching events, organised by Takako, that took place off the coast of Japan throughout 1998.

Shizuko and I left before these took place. After the playshops at Ikoi-no-sato we set off on a new adventure to visit Dr Hiroki Kozawa and the patients at his clinic in Hekinan City in Aichi Prefecture.

Chapter 19
Dr Kozawa's Clinic

Dr Hiroki Kozawa, who was born in Hekinan City in 1949, graduated in 1974 from the Toho School of Medicine in Tokyo, where he specialised in gastro-intestinal surgery. Ten years later he returned home to take over the clinic that was owned and run by his parents, both of whom were physicians. Once fully in charge of the clinic Dr Kozawa turned away from allopathic medicine and adopted an Oriental method of treatment, based upon macrobiotic diets. These he combined with the use of EM-X (effective micro-organisms – formulation X), a form of therapy being developed by Dr Teruo Higa, Professor of Agriculture at the University of Ryukyus, with whom Shizuko had close connections. I had first met Dr Kozawa in Zurich in 1998 where he explained his methods to me.

'My method of treatment is the biological and physiological application of Oriental philosophy and medicine, a dialectical conception of the infinite universe,' he told me. 'Macrobiotics is 5000 years old and shows the way to happiness and health.'

Dr Kozawa said he viewed the symptoms of his patients as indicators of the need for change, both in their way of thinking and eating. Instead of 'attacking' their diseases with surgery, he encouraged his patients to work with him to find a cure. In place of being passive recipients they became active participants in their respective treatments.

Dr Hiroki Kozawa met Shizuko and I off the train and ferried us across the flat Japanese landscape to his clinic. To reach his living accommodation we towed our suitcases through a garden bursting with organic produce. Cackling chickens scuttled before us like flying fish before the bow of a ship under way. The chickens were especially bred to provide fertilised eggs, not meat, for the treatment of anaemia in cancer patients.

Dinner was served in the kitchen. The good doctor detected the momentary arch of my eyebrow when I did not recognise the food, apart from the brown rice, which was placed before me. With considerable delight he identified each of the mysterious ingredients and assured me of their antioxidative properties. I lavished appreciation on the therapeutic benefit I felt sure I was deriving from the bottle of excellent French wine which he produced, an item I was given to understand that was not included on the clinic menu.

Our genial host had an immense sense of fun. I wondered how much of the Patch Adams school of medicine, which embodies the principle that laughter itself is healing, he carried over to the treatment of his patients.

Because of the differences between his methods of treatment and those of the Western school of medicine that had been instilled in me, I asked our generous host to run through the overall philosophy of his approach to disease which he saw as dis-ease, especially cancer. He told Shizuko and I that he viewed the presence of carcinomas as 'body messengers' that he had to work with to bring about change. Cancers, he said, concentrated oxidative and poisonous substances. They should not be attacked and killed. Instead, patients should stop eating sugar and fat etc and thereby cleanse their bodies. When this happened the cancers no longer had a role to play, and disappeared.

Thus the first thing Dr Kozawa did for a patient who presented with cancer was to impose a strictly controlled diet, which he claimed also clarified the patient's aura. Dr Kozawa also asked those in his care if they had a mission in life. This he insisted was important, because it gave them a reason for living.

Dr Kozawa also outlined what he described as the need for cancer patients to attain 'more spiritual energy values'. These, he said, were reached with joy and creative activities.

'Am I right in saying that, in effect, you are creating an environment in which your patients are healing themselves?' I asked.

'Exactly,' he replied. 'When I have done that I am no longer necessary. My patients become my teachers.'

'And you tell your patients that?'

'Yes.'

Like most Japanese, Dr Kozawa did not view death in the same way that most Western doctors do – to be prevented at almost all cost. In his view death should not be approached with fear, but with joy, as the moment of peaceful transition to another dimension. Part of his job was to help each of his patients attain a level of spiritual peace so they could pass smoothly on the journey into their next existence.

After dinner those patients who were capable of leaving their beds were summoned to congregate in the vestibule of the clinic which was to serve as my lecture room. Most of my generation still perceive dolphins as fish which are reptiles and lay eggs. The enlightened ones know that dolphins are warm-blooded aquatic mammals that gave birth to live young. As my mostly elderly audience assembled, I pondered on how many of them were in the latter category. Not many.

I tried to put myself in their position. How would I, as an ill person, feel about being dragged out of bed in the evening to be given a talk in an utterly incomprehensible foreign language about a fish. The answer. Not happy.

I did not understand a single word of what Dr Kozawa said when he introduced me. Whatever it was, it achieved the impossible. It changed the expressions on the faces of my audience to ones of even greater gravity.

I already knew from my ICERC experience that if my tongue-in-cheek jokes were translated literally into Japanese they would be taken seriously and would have exactly the opposite effect to that intended. So I was denied the most effective method I have of winning over an audience. Laughter. But I did have Shizuko. She could tell jokes in Japanese. And so the Anglo-Japanese equivalent of the Morecambe and Wise duo went into action with me taking the serious Ernie Wise role, and Shizuko putting her own unique Eric Morecambe twist to what I said.

My audience did appear to move a little more briskly when they left than when they arrived. 'Is that just because they are anxious to get back to their beds?' I wondered.

Dr Kozawa said he judged the evening to be a great success. Later events were to show that those present absorbed more than I was aware. But just how much influence my talk had had on one member of the audience, for whom it was a life-changing experience, was not revealed until it was time for Shizuko and I to leave the clinic the next morning.

One aspect of the dolphin way of life which I feel I should emulate but can never ever achieve, is that they don't carry baggage. In their world passports are not needed. Their brains can carry the images that I record with my camera. They don't need changes of clothes. They are always ready for a game and are therefore free to enjoy the moment, uncluttered by possessions.

I am the opposite of this. I cannot go anywhere without excessive amounts of luggage. Even a day trip to London invariably requires that I have to sit on my briefcase before I can snap shut the locks. When it comes to overseas travel I excel in the ability to take with me so many cases that even a Sherpa would wince at carrying them for fear of getting a hernia. However, as this disease is incurable it is not unknown for me to accept kind offers by would-be porters of either sex, who, in a moment of sympathy, offer their services. When

Shizuko and I arrived at the Kozawa Clinic a strong female nurse, well versed in lifting patients in and out of bed, appeared from nowhere and offered to hump cases to our quarters. When the time came to leave the Kozawa Clinic, however, I was faced with a different situation.

One of Dr Kozawa's patients who was half my size, and looked as if he could barely manage to support the weight of his own frail body, let alone my heavy suitcases, insisted on taking on the role of porter, not just at the clinic, but all the way to Kyoto and then on to the airport. I explained to him, via Shizuko, that although I might not look like a weight-lifter, after years of practice I could in reality manage to carry my cases to wherever they had to go. But all my protestations were to no avail. When we set off for the railway station, en route for Kyoto, he settled in beside me, to be close at hand whenever I needed him.

On the long train journey to Kyoto, Shizuko translated what my companion, who was still sitting next to me, was communicating.

'He says he is a humble school teacher. Throughout his life he has never achieved much. Just before he was due to retire he had a serious heart attack. Everyone thought he was going to die. So he collected his insurance. Then he heard about Dr Kosawa and his life started to change,' said Shizuko. 'He has been at the clinic for the past four months. He says he never knew anything about dolphins before he heard you speak. He is amazed by what you have said about them. You and the dolphins have given him strength. Normally he doesn't get up until late. There is no need to do so. When you mentioned last night that Dilo had a mission he realised he had a mission too. That is why he got up at 5.00am this morning. To make sure that he would be there to help you. He said because of you he feels strong again. Strong enough to start his mission.'

'I'm very flattered,' I said 'but I don't want him pegging out on us with another heart attack.'

I don't know what Shizuko said to our companion but he smiled in reply. I interpreted this as an expression of agreement.

At the temple in Kyoto, Kokyo Konoe had put out the word that Shizuko and I were in town and would be putting on a show there that evening. His advance publicity worked well and the room was nicely full of people, one of whom, Takako Suzuki, who spoke a little English, made a point of introducing herself to me. She had an autistic son and was keen to hear more about Eve. She handed me a laconic note in English. *I want to build work place and a relax house for handicapped peoples. I decided name for it. That's Dilo house! from Takako Suzuki.* I introduced her to my luggage carrier, Michio Matsumaga, and they were soon engrossed in conversation. I later found out that she told him her dream was to find a place, full of dolphin energy, to which she could take her son and others like him.

I asked Michio if he would like to say a few words during the course of the evening to the assembled multitude. He agreed. It was like releasing a captive bird from a cage. At first he was a little cautious and apprehensive. Then, when he discovered his freedom, he soared.

The man we parted company with the next day after he had escorted Shizuko and I to Osaka Airport was not the man who had reluctantly dragged himself along to hear a talk by a foreigner about a fish at the Kozawa Clinic. He was a man transformed. I know this because months later I received a long letter in Japanese from Michio. Shizuko kindly translated the letter, word for word, into a tape recorder.

In his letter Michio gave me a potted autobiography. He explained how he had harboured a dream to help children who find it difficult to learn and were disruptive in class. The dream had got progressively stronger during his 37 years as a teacher, but remained unexpressed. When he had his heart attack it was abandoned completely. It was time for him to pass on, or so he thought.

From what Dr Kozawa had told us over dinner I would not be surprised if he had subtly suggested to Michio that he needed a reason to stay alive. But the ex-teacher didn't realise it until I gave my talk in the clinic.

However, it was in the Dolphin Healing Centre in Kyoto, when Michio spoke to Takako Suzuki, that the precise nature of his mission suddenly became crystal clear. She wanted a house full of dolphin energy where people with mental problems could go. He, Michio Matsumaga, would create such a house. Indeed, he knew of just the place – an old farmhouse he had visited 20 years earlier, about 50 km from his home.

After parting company with us at the airport, Michio Matsumaga decided to leave the Kozawa Clinic and find the farmhouse. Which he did. When he reintroduced himself to the Nishimura family who owned it, he discovered that since his previous visit an autistic child had been born there. This was a sign. He had found the light. The parents of the autistic child offered him the house as a place where children could come to experience and learn about nature. In the spring nightingales sang from dawn to dusk. It was paradise. The farmer had changed to organic farming and had a spare piece of land. Michio organised a rice-planting festival and raised 50 volunteers. Over two weekends they brought the field into production.

At this stage of the translation Shizuko produced a photo she had taken. It showed Michio illuminated with rays of golden light walking through a field of soft yellow-green vegetation. She had encouraged Michio to follow his mission and had joined him on the farm during one of the weekends.

'The children had an absolutely wonderful time planting rice and playing in the mud,' she said.

The school teacher's interest in skiing was also rekindled. He visited Switzerland.

In his letter Michio referred to the help received from one of Shizuko's special friends, Motoko, who is also a healer.

'Motoko-san came to my hotel in Zurich. She gave me kiko energy. With her help I went up into the Swiss Alps, something I would never have done before,' he enthused.

On 11 December 1999 I had a phone call from a very excited Shizuko. She told me that she was at Schipol Airport, in Holland, on her way to Japan. Just before she left her house a fax came through from Michio addressed to both of us.

'It's amazing,' she said, barely able to control her excitement. 'Michio has become a new man, full of youth. He is so completely changed. He is a Japanese Bill Bowell!'

Shizuko said she would buy a tape recorder and translate the letter for me during the long flight to Japan.

True to her word she posted the tape to me on her arrival in Japan. When it reached my house a few days later it was like an unexpected Christmas present. In it Michio told how miracles had continued to happen to him. Now 62, he was back at work.

'My youth started again when I was 60,' he wrote.

After the seriously ill teacher was touched by dolphins during my talk at the Kozawa Clinic, he took part in a peace march from Tokyo to Hiroshima, where the first atomic bomb was dropped in World War II, walking 200 km in ten days. He had climbed to 2900 metres in what he called the Japanese Alps. On a trip to Norway, Denmark and Sweden in August 1999, Michio had run 10 km every day.

However, taking precedence over these personal physical triumphs was his ongoing progress with the 18-year-old autistic girl on the organic farm and with what Shizuko translated as 'school refusing children', in other words children who, for various reasons, would not go to school. Michio involved these emotionally disturbed pupils in activities from planting to harvesting. He also wanted to interest them in sport. But no sports centres would allow them in. Just when he was about to give up he found a back-street gymnasium where they could bounce on the trampoline and participate in health gymnastics. Michio was especially pleased with the progress of one recalcitrant child who he taught to ski and swim. He explained how he used the Dilo stories to encourage him.

'Now I am a young man again,' Michio concluded. 'And I want to help many, many more children like this.'

As I listened to the tape I pondered on how, in their own extraordinary way, the dolphins had enabled this modest man to overcome his heart problems. In addition the spirit of the dolphins had given him a new zest for life and the prospect of fulfilling a faded dream.

In a completely different way, the dolphins also enabled me to re-connect with a dream had I harboured since childhood – to unravel the mystery of Atlantis. A trip to the Bahamas was to offer me an opportunity to explore the myth of the lost city.

Chapter 20
The Stress Solution

In recent years stress has grown steadily with our standard of living. A certain amount of stress is necessary to stimulate the creative juices that make life worth living. But too much stress leads to all kinds of problems, none more so than in personal relationships. And this was an area in which I felt dolphins could play a healing role.

'Could swimming with dolphins provide an antidote for the stresses of modern day living?' was the question I posed myself.

When Rebecca Fitzgerald told me she was going to run a Dolphinswim programme from Bimini in the Bahamas, I decided to put this theory to the test. However, I had another reason for wanting to go to Bimini. There is an offshore reef, the Bimini Road, which is reputed to lead to Atlantis.

The myth of Atlantis, an ancient civilisation lost beneath the sea, intrigues me. What kind of cataclysm could have made an entire city disappear without trace? Who lived there? Did they associate with dolphins? And if so, do dolphins still carry some lingering memory of the people or the place?

In the Bahama Archipelago there are places called Blue Holes which are literally just that. They are holes that disappear like mine shafts deep beneath the sea bed. Some of them contain amazing arrays of stalactites and stalagmites. I know because I have dived in one of them. Such formations are created by evaporation of dripping water. For this to occur they must, at sometime, have been above sea level. This is irrefutable evidence that in the geological past the landscape of the Bahamas must have been very different to the collection of low lying islands we know today. This being so, was Atlantis, if it ever existed, sited in the Bahamas? Could the Bimini Road lead to the lost city? There was a way to find out. Go there.

Shizuko and I met at Miami Airport in August 1997 and arrived on Bimini in style – by seaplane. Fifteen minutes after splashdown we had cleared immigration and customs and were rattling along the road, swerving around the biggest potholes, to the Bimini Bay Club. Standing like a giant wedding cake on its own peninsula, surrounded by the gently waving palms, the building with its rambling, idiosyncratic architecture, greeted us as if it were an old friend. In the dining room a large bay window brought the outside vista into the room.

'This is a dream set in a dream,' exclaimed Shizuko, her eyes, as well as her words, expressing her delight.

Outside the window, about half a mile offshore, sit the Three Sisters – three tiny coral islands, dark against the surrounding azure sea. Occasionally a cloud of foam bursts beside one of them. White froth creams over the surface and is gone. The sea continues to dash against the rocks waiting for the seventh wave to infuse it with sufficient energy to erupt once again. Nearby, beneath the sea and invisible to us, lies the Bimini Road – a mysterious formation of rocks which some say is the road to the lost city of Atlantis.

Further out to sea there is another road along which the dolphins roam like strolling players. Nobody knows where it comes from or where it goes. It is an invisible road. The dolphins move its location every day. But the word is that if you sail straight out to sea from the Three Sisters you will intersect the Dolphin Road. And when you do that, if the dolphins are in the right mood, then you will have an experience that will change your life forever.

But exactly what is the nature of that change? What really happens to make meeting a dolphin such a profound experience for those with autism or suffering from chronic depression? Can the magic that worked for them be used to relieve the multifarious medical and social problems that arise from the stressful world into which we are being inexorably drawn?

As we watch the sun go down I ask Shizuko if she has seen a green flash at sunset.

'What is the green flash? I know not anything of it,' she responds.

I explain that I have often looked, but have never seen it. At that precise moment the sun dips beneath the distant horizon. As it does so, a shaft of bright yellow-green light, swift as a lightening flash, lights the line between the sky and the sea and is gone. It is the elusive green flash.

'This is omen,' says Shizuko. 'I think many surprising things are going to happen here on Bimini.'

As the light fades we venture forth to find Rebecca and her husband Mike who have just sailed across from Miami on board their boat *Echo* which will also be their base for the next two weeks. On board we have a rowdy reunion helped along with rum punches which slip down effortlessly and seem to have little effect on me, although they do make the others noisier. When I stand up, however, I discover my legs have turned to rubber.

Most of the participants in the Dolphinswim party arrive on the seaplane next morning. Having spent an entire day on the tiny island, Shizuko and I regard ourselves as old hands. We all gather at one of a group of condominiums (known as 'condos') which are to be occupied by Rebecca's 18 guests. I share a room with Koji Ishiwara, a young man from Japan. Shizuko's room-mate is from Holland. It is a multi-national gathering. Everyone speaks English. Rebecca tells us that she reckons the best time for dolphin encounters is in the late afternoon. Each day at about 4.30pm we set out to sea, always prepared for the option that the dolphins might not come to join us; but most times they do.

I am an early riser. The habit stayed with me on Bimini. One morning I awoke and peered out. The sky was dark with clouds. Lightning was zigzagging down into the sea. I love storms. I find the crack of lightning and the rumble of thunder immensely exhilarating. Leaving my room-mate fast asleep I crept out and went for a swim. The heaving sea was grey. Lightning fired down around me. This was what it must have been like when life first appeared on our planet. The water was charged with incredible energy. I pulled off my trunks and held them in my hand. I wanted to be totally at one with the force of nature. I knew it was madness. Suddenly I was in the middle of a squall. The rain lashed down in torrents. I shouted at the sky. I was jubilant. I wanted to feel it. I don't think I have ever felt more alive than at that moment.

The squall passed. I pulled on my trunks and swam back to the beach where a small group, astounded by my stupidity, were anxiously awaiting my return. It was time for breakfast, and more unplanned dramatic entertainment. We were all tucking in when Mike shouted 'Hey, look guys – a waterspout!'

A heavy cloud bank was moving towards us. From its base, first one, then two dark fingers appeared. They pointed directly down to the sea. Immediately beneath them were patches of white water.

'They are tornadoes,' said Mike. 'They're sucking up water from the sea.'

We dropped our knives and forks and ran outside. One waterspout moved off and disappeared. The other was moving towards us. We watched mesmerised. It was coming straight for us. Soon we could see a huge dish of white foam on the sullen grey sea. From it, like the twisting trunk of a giant palm tree, rose a tube of swirling water that soared skywards, until it disappeared into the clouds.

I could understand why they were called twisters.

Closer and closer it came. The patch of tormented white

water beneath it advanced inexorably towards us. When it was 100 metres off, we rushed inside the house and watched through the windows, spellbound, exhilarated, and then petrified, as it made its final approach. One person, however, didn't come inside. My courageous room-mate, Koji, stayed out. We waited for the tornado to strike. By now the spout was about 20 metres from the beach. Then suddenly it veered to our right. The casuarina pines suddenly came to life. They flung their branches hither and thither, dancing in the circular wind which was now heading towards the road leading to the house in which we were cowering. Koji ran down the sandy lane to intersect the path of the tornado. He dropped on his knees. Then it hit him. The young man disappeared in a whirlwind of sand and flying pine needles. Within a second the tornado had passed and continued its journey into the mangroves behind us. Koji stood up, dusted himself down and trotted back towards the house. Everyone applauded. Spattered with dust and dark, dead pine needles, he treated us to one of his endearing, self-effacing smiles and said, 'I am happy person.'

We all clapped and returned to breakfast.

As the morning was free and the weather appeared to be clearing up, I suggested to Koji that we should snorkel the half-mile or so to the Three Sisters. When we set off the sea was relatively calm but was getting up a little. After we had inspected the life around the islands I said that it seemed a pity to come so far and not progress for another half-mile to the reef known as Bimini Road, which I had yet to see. There was one small problem. Locating it. The Three Sisters were clearly visible because they could be seen from the surface. Our new destination was completely submerged. We would have to look for it. As we headed in what I hoped was the direction of the road to Atlantis the weather took a turn for the worse. Considerably worse in fact. This didn't worry me at all. Going up and down on the waves in a heavy sea is not uncomfortable. I had done it many times. When we rose on the top of a wave I got a glimpse of the shore by which I was trying to navigate. When we were in a trough the shoreline disappeared altogether. During our long swim we scanned the sea bed through our facemasks, but could see no sign of the reef we were searching for. The above-water visibility started to get worse as the weather continued to deteriorate further. With a strong, young companion I had no fear for his safety, or mine. Unfortunately this lack of concern on my part was not shared by those on shore who could no longer see us. A search and rescue operation was mounted. Mike launched a boat and set out in the now raging sea to see if he could find us. When we crested a wave I saw the boat. I took off a fin and waved it in the air so he could see us. As he coasted up I shouted. 'Mike, I can't find the Bimini Road, can you tow us to the spot.'

Mike was completely taken aback. 'Everyone on the shore thinks you're drowning.'

I had neglected to take into account the fact that the people in the group were not a team of experienced divers who were familiar with treacherous and testing conditions which had been my training ground in the cold and often wild seas around the coast of Britain. 'Oh, dear,' I replied realising what a gaffe I had made. 'In that case you had better tow us back to the beach.'

The cheers and hugs Koji and I received when we staggered out of the jaws of death and up the beach almost compensated for the disappointment of not finding the road to Atlantis.

The existence of the Bimini Road was first recorded in 1968. The site was photographed in 1969 by Dimitri Rebikoff who took a series of underwater pictures which he pieced together like a mosaic. After diving the site and examining the photographs, archaeologists put forward the hypothesis that the blocks were hewn in situ from the solid coral base in a manner similar to the other ancient submerged harbours surveyed in the Mediterranean and elsewhere, constructed during the Bronze Age over 3000 years ago.

If this is true, then it throws an interesting light on the earliest human inhabitants of Bimini. Could they have been related to the Mayans and the Incas, evidence of whose architectural prowess and extraordinary civilisations abound in

South America? It was thoughts like this that hardened my resolve to inspect the Bimini Road.

To prevent a repeat of the previous fiasco Mike made sure we stopped off at the submerged reef on our next boat trip to see the dolphin. When we arrived I repeatedly snorkelled down the 5–7 metres to the flat, roughly rectangular tables of native limestone to examine them. I swam the full length of the Bimini Road several times. I guessed it was about 100 metres long before it disappeared under the sand. Here and there it sprouted corals that swayed back and forth in the gentle swell. The tropical fish were not profuse, but they were diverse, and I recognised numerous familiar friends.

As I snorkelled along, peering down, two nurse sharks appeared. They cruised languidly across the sea bed towards the reef beneath me. They summoned enough height to traverse it; then, still finning slowly and deliberately, they descended once more to the expanse of ribbed sand beside the Bimini Road. With effortless sweeps of their tails, the two strollers continued their journey in a straight line. Within moments they disappeared into the distance as silently as they had come. I had filmed sharks in many parts of the world and I knew nurse sharks to be completely harmless. For me it was like seeing two friends out for a stroll. I later explained this to one of my fellow snorkellors who, on seeing the sharks, had shot back to the boat at an impressive speed.

What turned out to be our best encounter with the dolphins on this trip happened after we had made a couple of runs out to sea and back without success. Our hopes of contact were beginning to fade when, from out of nowhere it seemed, a small posse of dorsal fins zoomed across the surface towards us. The atmosphere on the boat changed immediately to one of joy and excitement. The dolphins first circled the boat and then remained near the bow, shooting through the water just ahead of us like silver arrows. They rose and fell in the flying spray and constantly changed positions. Sometimes three were in line, as if formation flying. Then one would drop back as another curved in to take his or her place. The newcomer might weave from side to side before accelerating ahead and looping away. The joy and energy of the dolphins was palpable.

When it was time to get into the water, there was a scramble to put on fins, masks and snorkels. The moment had come to enter the world of the dolphins. Some went in boldly, striding into the sea from the boat's water-level platform. Others sat on the platform with their feet dangling in the water before sliding in. Once in, everyone finned towards the dolphins, which were swimming around excitedly, like children in a playground. Indeed, that's exactly how it was for all of us, humans and dolphins alike.

The dolphins followed Mike as he swam rapidly down towards the bottom. When he reached the sandy sea bed about 8 metres down, he pointed his video camera upwards to film the snorkellors spread out on the surface. The dolphins corkscrewed around him, jostling with one another for a position in front of his lens. When he drifted slowly back upwards the dolphins continued to envelop him. Then they broke off and played amongst the swimmers.

The least experienced members of the party just floated on the surface, peering down through masks and breathing through their snorkel tubes. The dolphins flitted from one to the next, leaving each person feeling specially honoured by a dolphin visit. Others followed Mike's example and dived into the depths.

Kathy from New Mexico watched her daughter Kristin swim gracefully down to meet a mother dolphin and her one-year-old baby. Not that the youngster was that small. Indeed the young female was already about two-thirds the size of her parent. The mother was covered with a generous stippling of black and dark grey spots on her silver-grey body, whereas her offspring had none. The common name of the delightful mammals who were sporting with us was, appropriately, spotted dolphins. Not until they are a year old do the dolphins get their first spots. After that the spots become progressively more numerous. Thus each dolphin's appearance changes continuously. When they reach old age many of the spots merge, giving senior citizens a very attractive mottled appearance.

The young female dolphin separated from her mother and sped towards Kristin who was spiralling down in a way that invited play. The youngster responded and swam past Kristin trailing one of her pectoral fins, or flippers, along the swimmer's body. Still staying below, Kristin switched to the dolphin stroke moving both fins in unison. Then she swam upside down, facing the surface. Her view was now the surface of the sea spread out like a waving, semi-silvered sheet through which she could see the blue sky and white clouds. Into her vision came the young dolphin. As the dolphin glided between Kristin and the surface, it once again gently stroked the young woman's body with a fin. It was a magic moment of tender inter-species tactile communication, initiated by the dolphin. The mother dolphin, who was twisting and turning between other swimmers, was fully aware of what her offspring was doing. When Kristin surfaced for another breath the mother and baby left their human playmates and swooped towards one another. They slowed. Then, with fins touching, they gradually disappeared into the distant haze of the limit of our visibility. Moments later they re-appeared below us – this time playfully trailing their fins across the sea bed, leaving clouds of sand in their wake. Before it had settled, they separated and hurtled towards the surface to join the swimmers and the other dolphins.

Then, quite suddenly, the game was over. All the dolphins were gone – or appeared to have gone.

Everyone swam back to the boat and scrambled on board, happily exchanging accounts of their encounters. One person however remained in the sea.

'Look,' said Kathy, pointing to the last lone swimmer, 10 metres away from the boat. 'The dolphins have come back.'

Those on the afterdeck stopped towelling themselves and watched the solitary swimmer who was being escorted by two dolphins, one on each side, so close that they were touching her. Kathy knew that this person was hoping her trip to Bimini would help her come to terms with her own emotional problems. Now she was receiving the dolphin treatment for which she had come. Everyone on board recognised that this was a sacred moment, a moment of divine bliss, and respected it. Nobody attempted to get into the water. We all just stood and witnessed the event.

The spell was broken when two more dolphins, looking for action, re-appeared alongside. Soon we were all kitted up again and back in the sea. The boat moved off and circled around us. More dolphins joined in. Mike dived and was surrounded by a tangle of eight dolphins swirling around him. As he surfaced more dolphins rushed in. Then even more arrived. Like a gang of motorcyclists with engines roaring, they zigzagged amongst us. They were here, there and everywhere. Outnumbering the humans, the dolphins swooped down to the sea bed and then soared up again. The sea was alive with dolphins. Everyone was electric with excitement. We didn't know which way to look next. We estimated there were at least 30, but it was hard to tell exactly because they were moving so fast. It was like being in a dolphin snowstorm. Eventually the dolphins closed ranks and formed into a jostling column. They mingled briefly with a group of swimmers and then raced off down the Dolphin Road. Within seconds they had gone. We watched their dorsal fins vanishing into the distance. Then, as if to signal their appreciation of our company, one after the other, three dolphins rocketed out of the sea, spun in the air and dropped back with a splash before continuing on their way. In the west the piled cumulus clouds were set afire by the orange orb of the sun falling slowly into the heaving sea.

When it was time for Shizuko and I to leave Bimini, I had no doubt in my mind that everyone who came on the trip left as a different person. Our hearts were all opened by the dolphins. For some the emotional floodgates were released. The tears they shed carried away the stresses that were blocking the resolution of problems arising from powerful personal relationships. Once again I was utterly convinced that this was not solely due to the getting-away-from-it-all effect of having a pleasant holiday, although that undoubtedly contributed. The dolphins themselves had played a major role in stress relief.

Ever since the introduction of the internet I have pondered on the possibility that once again we are mimicking nature. Is there a vast natural repository of knowledge about everything that has happened to our planet? If so, how and where is this information stored?

Thoughts like this were running through my mind as I swum down onto the reef that reputedly leads to Atlantis. Have the rocks somehow absorbed the knowledge of their past history? If so, could the dolphins use their intelligence and close affinity with nature to retrieve that information, and even pass some of it on to me?

Of course I could not answer such questions, but of one thing I was absolutely sure when I left Bimini in 1997. I had the basis of a storyline for a new Dilo book, in which he would have his ultimate adventure. Dilo would discover Atlantis.

Chapter 21
The Remora and the Bull Shark

In 1998 Sally Galotti and I completed a book for an Italian publisher. It was entitled *Potere Magico di Dilo* (Dilo's Magic Power). In it Dilo finds himself embroiled in exciting escapades off an island with an active volcano. In the book the dolphin has a constant companion who literally sticks to him through thick and thin because she is a remora or suckerfish. I named her Rema.

At first my mental image of Rema was based upon the small dark fish stuck to the back of a dolphin named Dobbie I had filmed in the Red Sea in 1981. Sally, however, was not fenced in by such reality. She had never seen a live remora and she let her imagination run riot. Rema's size and flamboyance grew with each successive creative stroke of Sally's airbrush and pens. The image of Rema she eventually showed me was the piscatorial equivalent of a flamenco dancer.

At first the scientist inside me was slightly resistant to the colourful, swirling finned character that was taking such a prominent role in Dilo's life. But my token resistance was soon dispelled. I was writing stories for children of all ages wasn't I? Walt Disney had set a precedent. He had turned a mouse, normally regarded as vermin, into a lovable cartoon character that was absolutely nothing like a real-life rodent. So why shouldn't we do the same thing with a fish that was regarded as a parasite? Also I felt that Rema might demonstrate to children, especially the 'no-hopers', that even animals seen as lowly by humans had attractive qualities and that their lives could be transformed if they tagged on to a dolphin – albeit a fictional one.

Sally loved Rema from the start. The more the character of the strange fish with a suction pad on her head developed, the more extravagantly stylised Sally's illustrations became. Sometimes she couldn't contain her enthusiasm. Sally would bubble with excitement and laughter when describing her latest creation to me over the phone from her studio in Milan.

When Sally and I agreed to join Rebecca on Bimini in 1999 I told my artist colleague that the chances of encountering a real-life Rema were remote.

Our base was Marlin Cottage where Ernest Hemingway wrote *Islands in the Stream*. His macho attitude to the underwater world posed an interesting contrast to my own. Knowing the way things work out for me, I suppose I shouldn't have been surprised at the events that took place on our first full day on the island. But I was. I recorded what happened in a rarely kept diary.

3 May 1999. It is Bank Holiday Monday back at home. We leave the jetty at 3.45pm and set off for our first dolphin swim – everyone is expectant. Skipper Melanie, tall, blonde, statuesque, gives the briefing. We head out to sea – no dolphins – we head back – no dolphins – we head out to sea again – no dolphins. Rebecca warned us this might happen. We make the last run and there they are. A baby jumps alongside. It has something stuck to its back. 'Horace, Horace,' squeals Sally, her eyes aglow. 'Do you see the suckerfish?'

Sally lies outstretched on the foredeck looking down into the sea as instructed by Melanie. Beneath her the baby dolphin is weaving from side to side, riding the bow wave. Sally can see the remora clearly. The dolphin looks up at Sally. For a short time, that will last forever in Sally's memory, the two are locked in eye contact. Sally's eyes flood with tears. Sally, who has been kitted up in her new wetsuit since we set off over two hours ago, must have been disappointed not to see the dolphins. But now it has happened she jumps into the sea and has a close-up view of the remora. It is different to the one I saw in the Red Sea. This suckerfish is colourful – a very attractive yellow and pink. When she comes out Sally is overjoyed that the remora she has been observing close-up is not just hanging on. The remora, now named Rema, was twisting around, almost as if it was dancing a jig. Did it sense Sally's presence and excitement?

The dolphins have not let Rebecca down completely, but our brief encounter is soon over. Nonetheless, everyone is happy. This is the first day. There will be more opportunities. The sun is setting. We head back for base.

'The dolphins have shown us once again that we are not in control,' I comment to the group. Then, to prove my point, just before we turn into the channel that leads to the dock, there is a group of spotted dolphins, close inshore, where they have never been seen before. We have been miles out to sea to look for them. And here they are, very close to the land. Nearly everyone goes overboard and has a wonderful time in the dusk. Sally and I stay on board and watch.

Then quite suddenly the dolphins are gone. We all look for them. The sea is flat. There is no way we can fail to see them when they surface. There are youngsters with them who come up frequently to breathe. But they have all vanished into thin air – or thick blue water

– whatever. There is absolutely no sign of them at all.

'How can they do that?' I ask.

'Perhaps they are non-corporeal bodies,' suggests fellow dolphin enthusiast Sara Charnos who amongst other things writes scripts for the TV series *The X Files*.

'What do you mean?' I ask.

'They have just turned into spirit,' she replies.

Wow, what a thought. 'Can dolphins turn from spiritual beings into physical beings and vice versa?' I ask myself. It could explain a lot of mysteries. But who but a boat-load of gullible, non-sceptics would even consider such a proposition? The week has started well.

The next entry, made a few days later, reflected the diversity of topics covered in the optional group get-togethers we had each morning in the balmy shade of a tree overhanging the verandah of Marlin Cottage.

At the playshop on day three, Rebecca made a remark that may be the key to dolphin healing. She said 'By giving us unconditional love the dolphins teach us how to give love. The love they give us grows like a plant, getting ever bigger. Then it is there for us to give to others, regardless of who they are. When we walk in love, disease (dis-ease) flows away.'

This was followed by a page penned in a completely different hand. It was a personal account by Eve Oxford Smith of her feelings when her dog was hit by a car and killed. It also recounted a legend which revealed how, long before I pontificated on the subject, the natives of North America knew that dolphins could help humans through the emotional stress of losing a dearly loved animal companion.

When we lose animals we love, their spirits move to the Rainbow Bridge where they wait for us. Then, when our spirit is ready, it travels to the Rainbow

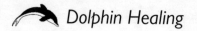

Bridge to join all our pets . . . Together, we then cross
the bridge to the Blue Dolphin Island where we live
together through eternity.

The next entry was in my own writing.

8 May 1999. *The day I was stalked by a large bull
shark.* This is the 'free day' between two Dolphinswim
groups. As the sun starts to set I decide to go
snorkelling on my own and head towards Entrance
Point which I guess is about half a mile away. It marks
the beginning of the channel that separates North and
South Bimini. If big fish are around, this is where they
will congregate. On my way I notice that the sergeant-
major fish are actively defending their nests, repeatedly
charging out at me and any other fish that passes by. I
see a stingray with a remora and the barracuda I have
watched previously in the same place. He hovers a foot
in front of me and I can see black lice scurrying over
his head. He needs a cleaning station. The rusting hull
of a ship, a casualty of a recent hurricane, is jammed
against the shore. The bronze propellor is still intact.
Onwards I swim. Five or six full-size tarpon, about 1.5
metres, very impressive fish, cruise between me and the
shore. I try to cut them off by swimming ahead but
having sussed my plan they accelerate into deeper
water. Then a huge shark cruises past. The underwater
visibility is cloudy. The sun is disappearing into a
massive grey cloud bank. The sea darkens. I turn round.
The shark is following me. I face it momentarily. It
stops. Then I change direction and swim towards the
shore. I turn round. The shark is still stalking me. Over
the years I have swum with hundreds of sharks and
filmed many of them. But this is the most menacing I
have ever seen. I guess it is about 2.5 metres long, dark
and with a big girth. I do not recognise it. It looks
mean. This is an oceanic shark – not a reef shark. The

bottom is littered with debris. I snorkel down and grab
a piece of aluminium tubing with bits of plastic bonded
to it. To me it is a tomahawk. Now I have a weapon
with which to face my stalker. I turn to face it again.
For a moment we both stay still, face to face. I brandish
my weapon. The shark turns and swims effortlessly
away. The ease with which the giant moves through the
water amazes me. No lashing of the tail. In fact it seems
to barely move its tail, yet it is travelling away from me
at a speed I could only match if I was swimming
frantically. It's gone. My attention is distracted by a
delightful group of cuttlefish. I move slowly forward so
as not to frighten them. I love cuttlefish. Their colours
are iridescent and change to match their surroundings. I
feel a tug on one of my fins. I turn round with a start.
It is Sally. Unbeknownst to me she has decided to
come for a late snorkel. 'I feel uncomfortable, Horace. I
feel there is danger.' My adrenaline level is still running
high. 'Have you seen that big dark shark?' I blurt out. It
is the wrong thing to do. Sally hasn't seen the shark or
the tarpon. She doesn't want to see the shark or the
tarpon and is not in the mood to hang around for a full
account of my encounter. The sky is getting darker by
the minute. 'Horace, I keep telling you, you must
become more spiritual'. 'What's that got to do with me
being stalked by a shark?' I ask, not seeing the
connection. She huffs at my lack of understanding and
turns back in the direction from which she has come.
'Hey, what about the cuttlefish, don't you want to see
them?' I don't need a reply. A pair of fins flashing at full
speed in a flurry of foam and disappearing into the
distance gives me my answer. Back at the house Mike
immediately recognises my description. 'It's a bull
shark,' he tells me. When I tell him how big it was he
dismisses it with the shrug of the master diver who has
been everywhere and seen everything. 'That's a tiddler,'
he tells me. 'Where I come from, we use sharks that size

for bait.' Not being taken seriously when you've just been given the evil eye by a monster shark is a trifle disconcerting. 'Just joking,' says Mike with an expansive grin. I hurry to the bookcase and fish out a book by Jerry Greenburg, a fellow underwater photographer who I knew years ago and whose shark photographs I admire. A picture immediately confirms Mike's identification:

> **Bull Shark** (*Careharinus leucas*) **A potential danger to swimmers**, the bull shark frequents inshore waters and sometimes enters rivers. A broadly rounded snout and heavy compact body distinguish this shark. The bull shark may grow to 3 metres.

So it wasn't an oceanic shark after all. I still have a lot to learn.

Despite the enormous number of divers who frequent Bahamian waters, as far as I know no shark attack on humans has ever been recorded. Indeed, I know of one dive operator who offers shark feeding as an optional extra activity. Even so, after Sally's response, I made no mention of the bull shark to the new group that arrived the following day for fear of spoiling the week for anyone of a nervous disposition.

The character of the new group was completely different to that of the previous week. Among those who disembarked from the seaplane was Shizuko. Shizuko's presence on Bimini gave me opportunities to have more debates with her on the differences between Eastern and Western attitudes to health. I found out, for instance, that not all of those present at Dr Nakagawa's 100th Natural Healing Seminar in Tokyo were actually ill.

Some were healthy and were there to experience an awakening to the 'joy of life', was how Shizuko explained it. With my Western way of thinking I interpreted this as preventative medicine in which the client, who is not a patient, receives a spiritual uplift that enhances the immune system.

'In the East, the job of the doctor is to keep you healthy. To do this you do not necessarily need lots of medical qualifications. Often the doctor is a wise person who has a knowledge of natural methods of maintaining health as well as knowing how to help those who are ill.'

'But what about people who are dying of cancer?' I asked.

'In the West we think of ill people as very unfortunate people. Unhappy people. Especially those with cancers.' Shizuko then proceeded to show me privately a series of gruesome close-up photographs of cancers taken at the Kozawa Clinic.

'But these are not unhappy people,' she continued, emphasising the word 'not'. 'Often they were not very happy people before they got their cancers. When they got cancer they saw the need for changes. And they became happy.' She showed me more photographs of patients with their wounds treated.

'It is part of their journey to becoming more spiritual. When they do this their cancers start to regress. Sometimes they disappear altogether.'

'What about those who don't respond?' I persisted.

'Some of them die. We all have to die. But they are happy when they pass on to the next world.'

This led us into Shizuko's interpretation of spirituality.

'Spirituality is not about religious conviction, or morality,' she explained. 'It is becoming aware of the spirit, of the joy of life which is in everything around us, especially dolphins.'

What Shizuko said reminded me of the final comments made by Auntie Pearl King, the Aborigine Elder, in her profound and powerful address at the opening of the ICERC Conference in Australia in 1997.

Spirituality is not about sitting isolated on a mountain top or in a monastery trying to transcend earthly distractions. It is not about sin or about feeling guilty. It is about living in life and finding the sacredness in everyday affairs. It is about everyday affairs including sacredness. It is about offering our joyful uniqueness to an embracing and accepting world. It is about honouring not only a paternal god but about honouring a maternal goddess as well. Australia and the rest of the world need a Great Mother to balance the Great Father. When we listen to Her, we are united with Mother Earth. That way the earth can guide us home to her own healing.

Even now I am still not sure that I fully understand what Shizuko was trying to explain to me. But what she said does make it clearer to me why dolphin healing is more readily accepted in countries like Japan, whose overall philosophies do not see prolonging life at all costs for as long as possible as the ultimate aim of the physician. It also added to my conviction that an intuitive understanding of the subtleties of the forces of nature was as important, if not more important, than a purely scientific approach in my quest for the essence of dolphin healing.

The dolphin encounters were somehow different during the second week. The most memorable encounter the second group had with dolphins took place on a day when I could not go out. I was on the jetty to greet the boat when it returned in the gloaming. Everyone on board was exploding with excitement at what had happened. They couldn't wait to tell me.

'Wow, you should have seen them Horace, they were mating and rearing out of the water whilst still locked together. It was amazing. Even when we all got into the sea the orgy continued. They liked us being there with them. The sea was teeming with dolphins making love. There must have been 40 dolphins at least.'

From the shore I had earlier watched a huge ominous, dark cloudbank creep towards the island. At the time I had wondered what was happening with the group out at sea.

'The sky turned black. Lightning flashed. The sea was filled with energy. It was amazing. Just amazing.'

This comment immediately brought back to mind my feelings when I had swum naked in the storm on a previous trip. I had felt there was an immense sexual energy in the water. Obviously the dolphins felt it too. And being completely uninhibited they acted without restraint in a joyous act of creation that infused the group of humans who had shared the sea with them.

Being humans, of course, everyone wanted a repeat performance the following day – and were genuinely keen that I should share a similar experience with them. However it was not to be, which made it all the more precious for them. It also showed how you never know what will happen next, and that the unexpected can occur at any time when you are in the company of a band of such free, strolling players as a group of spotted dolphins in the open sea.

At the end of the week we said our farewells outside Marlin Cottage. Rebecca was in tears. A delightfully crazy youngster, Suzie, an animal rights welfare worker, had stayed up part of the night composing a song. As we waited for the taxi to take us to the seaplane base she sat on the ground in the sunshine with the azure sea behind her and sang her song to us, accompanying herself on her guitar. When she finished she cried with emotion at the prospect of parting company with the group. Full of emotion she scooped up a handful of white coral sand and stuffed it into her pocket.

As we flew back to Miami, I wondered what was going on under the sea beneath me. What were the dolphins doing and thinking? Were they aware just how much love, laughter and sadness at leaving they had stirred up in us humans flying over them in a noisy seaplane? Or were they blissfully unaware of us, enjoying being totally free spirits and taking whatever came along, be it a bunch of humans, or another pod of dolphins, as part of the endless ribbon in their game of life?

Chapter 22
Dolphin-assisted Therapy

A healthy life is a high-wire balancing act. It is a miracle that we can stay there at all. During every second of every day of our lives, countless adjustments are being made to innumerable bodily functions, most of which we are totally unaware of. But if just one of them starts to go awry then illness can ensue, diabetes for example. To remain in good health our blood sugar levels must be kept within narrow limits despite the enormous variations in the quantity and nature of the food we eat. Another problem area is salt. We all need salt to survive. Yet too much taken over long periods brings problems and surprisingly little is lethal if a salt solution is injected. Food and salt are external factors over which we can exert direct control.

There are other factors over which we have little or no control. These are pathogens, foreign substances that enter our bodies and then have to be processed and eliminated. Viruses and bacteria are the two major culprits seeking to dislodge us from our high wire.

Bacteria are tiny organisms. They consist of single cells that are invisible to the naked eye but can be seen under an optical microscope. They are neither plants nor animals. Most of them are innocuous. Some are essential for breaking down food in the gut. Others, the pathogenic bacteria, can be dangerous. They kill living cells. If the conditions are right, bacteria can reproduce at a very rapid rate. Many can double their population in five minutes. Thus one bacterium can create four million in two hours. This explains why illnesses such as cholera can kill within 24 hours. Viruses are smaller and simpler than bacteria. They live inside cells and are so small they can only be seen with an electron microscope. After multiplying they burst out of their hosts, destroying the cells in the process. Viruses are responsible for a wide variety of medical conditions ranging from influenza and the common cold to AIDS.

Our bodies produce a whole range of processes for counter-attacking the invasion of bacteria and viruses. It is called the immune system.

The major weapons in our armoury are a variety of white cells (lymphocytes, leucocytes, mast cells and monocytes) that circulate in the blood. There are two types of lymphocytes. B-cells produce antibodies that fight bacteria and viruses from the outside. T-cells operate from inside infected cells.

When I disussed dolphin healing with therapist Rachel Charles she gave me a copy of her book, *Mind, Body and Immunity*. In it she elegantly describes the generation, function and control of these cells and other elements of the immune system. Rachel also points out that initially it was thought that the production of white cells was controlled at the sites, such as the bone marrow, where they originated. However, it was later discovered that immune responses can also be activated by neurotransmitters that originate in the brain. This lends plausibility to the notion that the mind, or the psyche, which is centred in the brain, can play a role in the management of medical problems, including those of viral or bacterial origin.

Of course, all who are involved in health from witch doctors to hospital consultants have long known that psychological factors can have a powerful influence on the onset and course of disease. Now that scientific evidence can be produced to support this obvious connection, a new branch of medicine with the pretentious title of psychoneuroimmunology (PNI), has come into being. Having jumped on board this bandwagon, I now propose that it is urged forward to make the next, even more blatantly obvious step, to PNH – psychoneurohealing. PNH recognises that psychological factors can play a key role not just in preventing diseases, but in curing them.

Because of what I do and who I am I meet countless people who are moved in some way by dolphins. I ask many of them why they feel so strongly emotional about dolphins. 'They make me smile'; 'They make me happy'; 'They make me feel good inside', are typical answers. But when I ask, 'How do the dolphins do it?' I never get a straight answer. A typical response is 'I don't know, they just do.'

After mulling over this question in my mind for more than 20 years I have come to the conclusion that deep down most of us have a love of our fellow humans and that dolphins concentrate this love. Unfortunately the behaviour of a small percentage of our race has buried that love under a layer of negativity. Sadly that layer of distrust, of antagonism, sometimes of outright hatred, is fuelled daily by news bulletins that feed us statistics on how many people have been killed or injured in a power struggle somewhere in the world. Nonetheless that love is there, and occasionally an event occurs that exposes this endearing side of human nature. The unprecedented and open outpouring of love that was expressed world-wide when Princess Diana was killed in 1998 is a case in point. It unequivocally demonstrated that most of us have love to give. We just have to find a channel to let it out. When we do that we heal ourselves.

As I stated in my introduction to this book, one of the purposes of this book is to show that dolphins can provide a channel through which love can flow, both from us and to us. The other is to unravel the mystery implicit in its title, *Dolphin*

Healing. This is a challenge I approach rather like a game of Cleudo in which a detective sets out to solve a murder mystery that takes place in a large house.

My workshops/playshops provide the settings. I am fortunate that these can and do happen anywhere in the world. Almost invariably they take place in interesting, and often attractive locations. Bimini for example. An advantage of Rebecca Fitzgerald's Dolphinswim programmes is that each one lasts for a week. This gives me adequate time to pose the riddle I want her guests to solve, namely: *how does dolphin healing work?* I then present the information and evidence we have to help solve the mystery.

One of the characteristics of dolphins is that there seems to be no rhyme or reason for the hearts they touch. Thus every person at a dolphin playshop can have a valid and valuable contribution to make. What eventually arises in these sessions depends to a considerable extent upon the make-up of the groups, who come from almost every conceivable walk of life, bringing with them an extraordinary array of talents and perspectives. We share experiences and discuss the impact dolphins have had on our lives. Sometimes we use music and art. Sometimes we do Dolphin Dreamtime, but most of all we learn from each other.

One of the most straightforward elements of the dolphin healing mystery is the dolphins themselves. What you see is what there is – which certainly cannot be said for most humans. With dolphins there is no duplicity. They don't wear clothes or make-up. The spotted dolphins of the Bahamas display their age like logos on teeshirts. The more spots there are, the older the dolphins. To my human eyes they become more beautiful with age. Although I have seen many geriatric dolphins, I have never met one that behaves as if it is old. Plenty of old folk still have the spark of youth inside them, but it is unable to burst into flame because of the burden of their aging bodies. Dolphins don't have to shuffle around in their later years, with a stick or frame for support. Their weight is entirely borne by water. With a light flick of the tail they can easily propel themselves with sufficient speed to catch a flatfish, or to frolic with a playful great-grandchild. So those seeking the holy grail of eternal youth can stop here. The dolphins have it. If you want it too, I suggest you try and fix it to come back as a dolphin in your next incarnation!

But to come back to the serious evidence gathering exercise. In our search for the source of dolphin healing, let's first look at a human and a dolphin together. We know that the dolphins spray us with sounds, few of which we can hear, but many of which could be having a physiological effect. These were apparent to Wendy Huntington (see p. 38) when the dolphins were around her. She said she felt like champagne. This supports the proposal made by Dr David Cole of the Aquathought Foundation in the US. He suggested that dolphin ultrasounds produce cavitation which stimulates the production of lymphocyte T-cells. These in turn selectively attack and destroy infected cells, including those hosting the AIDS or ME viruses.

During a visit to a fellow dolphin enthusiast Estelle Myers, at her home in the Blue Mountains of Australia in 1997, I was introduced to Dr Kay Distel, who was treating a child with profound behavioural and learning problems with sound. She introduced me to the work of a French physician, Dr Alfred Tomatis, who laid the groundwork for APP (audio-psychophonology) and has devoted much of his professional life to investigating how sound and speech play such a pivotal role in human emotions and behaviours, and then applying his findings clinically. Later I was contacted by a friend, Jill Robinson, who asked 'Do the sounds made by dolphins have a similar effect to the filtered sounds Dr Tomatis creates to facilitate the "sonic birth" of children, including those with autism, as described in his book *The Ear and Language*?'

I couldn't give her a categorical answer but it did make me even more aware of the immense complexity of the effects of sounds on the human body. I asked myself yet again how Dolphin Dreamtime has such an influence on so many people? And why did *Iruka No Uta* (The Dolphin Song) have such a powerful effect on my own ability to put my thoughts into words? Despite this, I felt the interaction of dolphin sound with humans was certainly not the full answer to the mystery of dolphin healing.

An acronym that has crept into common use in connection with dolphin healing is DAT – dolphin-assisted therapy. DAT is an appropriate way to describe the work of Dr David Nathanson, a very successful psychotherapist based in the US. I watched 'Dr Dave' as he is affectionately known by his patients, treating a brain-damaged adult and Bill, a two-year-old Down's syndrome child in 1989.

The therapy session took place in a completely relaxed atmosphere beside a dolphin pool in the Florida sunshine. Dr Nathanson showed his young patient an outline of a car painted on a wooden board. Dr Dave pointed at the picture and very clearly articulated the word 'car' several times. It was a game. When Bill tried to imitate the spoken word, Dr Dave gave the youngster every encouragement. When the boy finally uttered a word that sounded anything like 'car', Dr Dave was full of praise. 'Good boy. Good boy,' he enthused.

The picture board was then thrown into the pool. Bill was handed to his mother who was already in the water. A dolphin gave them both a tow. A smiling Bill was given more praise. The dolphin was rewarded with a fish by a trainer who had used hand signals and a whistle to instruct the dolphin on what manoeuvre to perform.

Dr Nathanson told me that he regards dolphins as adjuncts to his stimulation, reinforcement, encouragement and reward regimen. This was the treatment he proffered to patients whose neurological problems included needing to learn, or re-learn speech, muscular co-ordination and other functions which those of us who are healthy take for granted.

Skills, such as walking across a room, are normally under our voluntary control. They are acquired in early childhood and are maintained in later life, and depend upon the brain and the central nervous system triggering intricate successions of muscle contractions and relaxations. In the Nathanson method the role of the human therapist is accepted as an integral part of the treatment. The dolphin is there to assist the therapist.

When Bill Bowell, the man who first alerted me to the healing power of dolphins, was cured of depression there was no qualified therapist anywhere near him. A friendly dolphin in the open sea was the therapist, or appeared to be. There was, however, someone else present. Bill was accompanied by his wife Edna, who was terrified when she had to clamber down the harbour wall into the boat, but overcame her fear to be with him. Later, when watching from the boat, the dolphins gave Edna hope that her beloved Bill would recover. I didn't know this until she casually mentioned it several years later.

This previously hidden evidence, which I should have been alert to, but wasn't, does not invalidate the outcome. Bill is indeed completely better. He has become a healer himself although he does not make this claim. However, I now see that Edna, his wife, played a vital role in Bill's recovery because she brought another weapon into the mystery of dolphin healing. She brought love which she gave unstintingly to her husband.

Having identified love as the possible key, I then re-examined all of the other cases where I had seen remarkable improvements in those seeking help from dolphins. In every case there was a human carer who played a key role. And that carer added his or her own personal love to the unconditional love virtually every patient felt they were receiving from the dolphins.

Wendy Huntington's husband Tony was on board the boat when she had her miraculous experience with the dolphins and her symptoms of ME disappeared. Indeed it was Tony who stopped Rebecca calling Wendy back to the boat when she was alone in the water as dusk was falling. When Wendy eventually came back on board he was there to reinforce the experience and cherish and love her.

Reviewing the evidence of the dolphin healing mystery threw up another clue.

I discovered this other clue when reviewing the case of anorexic Jemima Biggs. When Jemima later visited Freddie, a friendly dolphin off Amble, in Northumberland, she cried for a whole day afterwards, something she had never done before. Her grief, for the death of her grandmother and other traumatic events in her life, was suddenly released in a torrent of tears. Then, like water from a spring, fresh feelings began to trickle into Jemima's consciousness. She began to love herself and recognise that others loved her too. She could freely receive love as well as give it. She was on the road to recovery. Indeed she got married and had two children.

The feeling that we are helpless and useless exacerbates medical problems. We all need to feel that our lives have some purpose. Helping a patient to find a task or mission in life is one way of fulfilling this need. An effective method is to encourage him or her to help others, in a totally unselfish way. Learning the joy of giving, without expecting anything back, in a society based upon a *quid pro quo* philosophy, is something we could all benefit from. Experiencing the joy of giving, therefore, is just one of the changes in attitude to life that should accompany dolphin therapy and enhance its efficacy. The more a patient can get away from a state of dis-ease, to one in which he or she can experience the exuberant joy of living and giving, which dolphins give out and we can feel when we watch them jump out of the sea for no better reason than the joy of being alive, the better are the chances of his or her recovery.

It has also become apparent to me during the course of my research that dolphin healing, as I perceive it, has many threads in common with other forms of alternative treatment, ancient and modern, each of which has its practitioners and advocates. This conclusion was brought into sharp focus for me by the Alternative Health section of *The Times* on 26 October 1999.

The first article to catch my eye was by Sally Morris on Ayurveda, which she claims is the world's oldest medical system, going back nearly 7000 years. 'Its name,' she writes, 'derives from two Sanskrit words – *ayus*, meaning life, and *veda* meaning knowledge.' Ayurveda is a highly skilled method of spiritual and physical healing which involves five years of study and one year at an Ayurveda hospital before a practitioner becomes properly qualified.

Ayurveda has helped countless patients over centuries, especially in India. It is a holistic approach which involves rethinking the way in which we lead our lives, including our diet – a method of treatment not inconsistent with that of Dr Kozawa in Japan.

Switching from the most ancient to the most modern, Susan Clark reported, in the same issue of *The Times*, on a radical treatment by the surgeon and qualified homoeopath, Dr James Colthurst. He uses a device called the Kosmed, which stands for cosmic medicine, and looks like a slim, black remote TV control. It sends a painless electrical impulse through the skin which stimulates the C-fibres of the neural network, resulting in the release of neuropeptides. These target the parts of the body needing repair, replicating natural, spontaneous, healing processes. Furthermore, the Kosmed switches off the process when the neuropeptides are no longer needed. Dr Colthurst's research produced dramatic improvements in sufferers of premenstrual tension and irritable bowel syndrome. Activation of the nervous system and subsequent release of neural hormones is consistent with the response of those whose medical problems have been magically ameliorated by dolphin therapy.

In between these two extremes was an article entitled: *Music: The new medicine* by Peta Bee. It described trials in which music helped patients overcome the trauma of surgery, and enhanced mental output in children. The songs of whales and dolphins are surely the music of the oceans. Thus an explanation, with some scientific back-up, can be advanced to further support the beneficial effects of listening to Dolphin Dreamtime.

From all of this it is apparent that dolphin healing is not a quick fix. It is a rung on a ladder. Furthermore, the dolphins need assistance to work their wonders. Thus dolphin healing is best coupled with conventional medicines, or with the so-called alternative or complementary treatments, such as reiki, reflexology, aromatherapy, crystal healing etc. Every case is different and requires its own special approach; intuition should not be neglected when looking for the best one. If one particular type of treatment feels right, then it probably is right. Professional counselling can play a useful role. But so too can just talking about a problem to a friend, or a sympathetic therapist, with dolphins playing a symbolic role.

There is, again, a common vital ingredient in all of the treatments I have reviewed. Yet it is seldom mentioned. And that, of course, is love.

So we have joy and love as the key elements in dolphin healing. I think we should also add hope to these. This combination of joy, love and hope pave the way to a positive, optimistic approach to medical problems stimulating the immune system responses which keep us on the high wire of life.

Think back to Dilo, and what happened when this mischievous dolphin swam into the hospitals and hospices of children dying of AIDS in Romania. Dilo carried with him the healing energy which dolphin images have radiated ever since they were used to decorate the Queen's bathroom at Knossos in Crete 3500 years ago. Added to this was the love given to the children by those who visited them, and those who cared for them.

This points to an extremely important corollary to dolphin healing. As well as the patients the carers too have their needs. These needs must be acknowledged, and satisfied, if the carers are to fulfil their roles, which are absolutely essential if dolphin healing is to be fully effective. So dolphin healing is also about giving hope to patients and those looking after them. With joy, love and hope present in abundance, the pathway to healing is open. We just have to follow it.

Into the New Millennium

The biggest force for change in the whole of human history, after the ability to create fire, was the discovery of electricity. Previously humans were aware of lightning. But the involvement of electrical energy, directly or indirectly in our everyday activities, from the manufacture of tools to powering cellnet phones, was utterly unforeseeable until Michael Faraday demonstrated the properties of electricity at the Royal Institution in London in the 1830s.

Without that new knowledge and understanding we could not possibly have conceived the role electricity plays in innumerable bodily functions, such as the beating of our hearts, which we can measure with an ECG (electrocardiogram).

But is there another power, yet to be discovered, which, like electricity, could have such an immense and incalculable influence on humans? I suggest there is. It is the power of life itself. It is in everything around us. We know it's there, but we don't understand it, at least I don't. I have referred to it as ki. Others call it prana or chi. Dr Nakagawa used it, and said everyone had an ability to do likewise. But for most people to do so requires a shift in consciousness which involves letting go of fear, seeing no boundaries and finding joy. It also requires an acknowledgement of other states of human existence apart from the purely physical, ie spiritual states.

This proposal begs further questions. Have the dolphins, unlike humans who have created tools and used them to investigate many aspects of physical reality, used their big brains to explore the realms of spiritual existence? Indeed are dolphins both physical and spiritual beings as some people have suggested? Is this related in any way to the ancient myths that dolphins carry the souls of the dead into the next world? And, if they exist, what are these spiritual levels of existence? How do we access them? Do we enter them when we go to sleep? If so could this explain why dolphins are more and more invading our dreams?

Only by asking such questions can we hope to reach a greater understanding.

Just like all of the other fields of scientific philosophical enquiry in which I have been involved, this journey through the healing power of dolphins has raised many new questions begging to be answered. Ever since Donald the dolphin made his first connection with me in 1974 I have witnessed an unprecedented rise in human–dolphin interactions. All the signs are that these will increase and the mystical bond between humans and dolphins will grow ever stronger. How this will affect human society as a whole in the future I find tantalising. Deep down I feel something really wonderful is going to happen. So as we humans step into another millennium I feel hopeful that we will be entering a new era of love and peace in the world. It's an exciting prospect, isn't it?

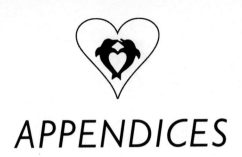

APPENDICES

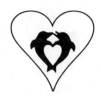

A Request

Each and every one of my books has a life of its own. I like to think of them as dolphins. They roam the world. Sometimes they are squashed into backpacks. You may encounter a dog-eared copy climbing the Himalayas, or in the Cairngorms. Smart ones cross the oceans in the cabins of cruise ships. Some are frequent fliers, soaring around the world above the clouds, while others nestle in the saloons of small boats, rocking to the swell at sea level. You may also find them rattling across the country in railway carriages or resting peacefully for a time on human laps in hospices. Some hide themselves in public libraries. Others have even been known to nestle among gold-leafed spines in royal bookcases. Some find themselves, like washed-up debris on the tideline, in the middle of heaps of clothes in teenagers' bedrooms. Wherever they are, that is where they are meant to be at that moment.

The question is, what happens to them next?

It is my view that books, like dolphins, should be free. They should bear the marks of their lives. They may have words written in them by hands other than mine. They may be tear stained. They may have coffee or cough mixture spilt on them. It doesn't matter. It adds to their character.

So, dear reader, I have a request.

I hope you have enjoyed the company of this book for a time. My request is that you now encourage it to 'swim away', as my friend Shizuko would say. Give it to a friend. Write a note and perhaps draw a picture inside the cover and put it in a school library where it can drift around, to who knows where, like a message in a bottle.

If you really can't bear to part company with it, can I suggest you purchase another copy (autographed if you wish) from International Dolphin Watch? It will be posted to you and all the proceeds will be used to help dolphins.

I also have a different suggestion to make to you. It is that you read bits of this book out loud to your children, your grandchildren, other people's children, to an elderly relative, to a blind person, or to someone with special needs. Don't be shy. It doesn't matter if you stumble over some of the words. The spirit with which you read them out loud is what matters. Your 'lipwords', as autistic Eve would call them, will carry the love of the dolphins in them.

Thank you.

The Dolphin Song

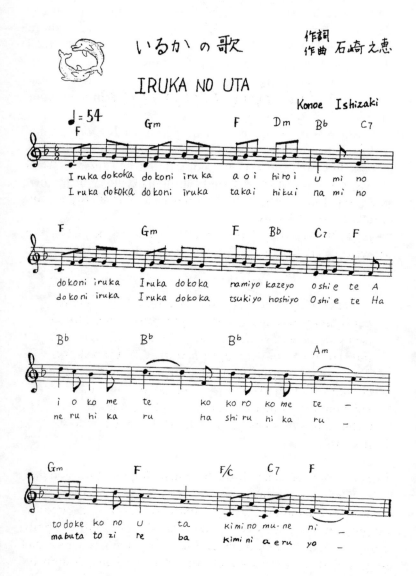

いるかの歌

作詞
作曲 石崎之恵

IRUKA NO UTA

Konoe Ishizaki

♩ = 54

F | Gm | F | Dm | B♭ | C₇

Iruka dokoka dokoni iruka aoi hiroi umi no
Iruka dokoka dokoni iruka takai hikui nami no

F | Gm | F | B♭ | C₇ | F

dokoni iruka Iruka dokoka namiyo kazeyo oshiete A
dokoni iruka Iruka dokoka tsukiyo hoshiyo Oshiete Ha

B♭ | B♭ | B♭ | Am

i o ko me te ko ko ro ko me te —
ne ru hi ka ru ha shi ru hi ka ru —

Gm | F | F/c | C₇ | F

todoke ko no Uta kimi no mu-ne ni —
mabuta to zi re ba kimi ni aeru yo —

178

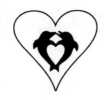

In Memoriam

I wish this book to be a memorial to Konoe Ishizaki, one of the co-founders of the Ki and Dolphin Healing Centre (see p. 69) who was born at the Myoren-ji Temple in Kyoto, and died there on 9 August 1999.

At 10.00pm on 26 November 1993, two weeks before the centre opened, Konoe had a vision in which the dolphins gave her the following message:

> Good evening! The fact is that you were born here to come and play a 'life' game. Be generous enough to play with anybody whom you encounter and also with those who say something nasty. You are all playfellows. There are humorous people and there are people who are not so humorous. Imagine that all of you are enjoying the game together. Some play a role of disliked person, some play a role of clown. Everybody has a role.

Konoe was a channel through which dolphin love and joy flowed. She and her husband Kokyo passed it on to those who came to the Dolphin Healing Centre. Konoe was inspired by dolphins in many ways. She wrote *Iruka No Uta* (The Dolphin Song) – see p. 178. Actually, she said the dolphins wrote the song, and that she was merely the channel. The question of copyright therefore did not arise. The song was free for anyone to use. For me, the melody has the timeless qualities of a traditional tune such as 'Greensleeves', or 'Danny Boy'.

I was deeply moved when Kokyo Ishizaki sent me, after his wife died, a mini CD of *Iruka No Uta*. It was packaged with typical Japanese delicacy and included a misty picture of his wife as a beautiful young woman beneath a lacy parasol.

With this tribute to his late wife, Kokyo included a letter in which he told me that despite the loss of his partner, and a certain resistance from the authorities, he would continue the work of the Ki and Dolphin Healing Centre.

One of Kokyo's wishes was that his wife's dolphin melody should float freely around the world carrying with it her message from the dolphins of peace, joy and love.

Selected Reading

Alpers, Antony, *Dolphins*, John Murray, 1970

Asaoka, Koji, *The Extraordinary Healing Power of Ki Energy*, Win Honest Planning, 1994

Carwardine, Mark, *On the Trail of the Whale*, Thunder Bay Publishing, 1994

Carwardine, Mark, with Erich Hoyt, R. Ewan Fordyce and Peter Gill, *Collins Whales and Dolphins*, HarperCollins, 1998

Charles, Rachel, *Mind, Body and Immunity*, Cedar, 1993

Cochrane, Amanda with Karena Catten, *Beyond the Blue*, Bloomsbury, 1998

Cousteau, Jaques-Yves, *The Silent World*, Hamish Hamilton, 1953

de Bergerac, Olivia, *The Dolphin Within*, Simon and Schuster, 1998

Deguchi, Kyotaro, *The Great Onisaburo Deguchi*, Aiki News, 1998

Doak, Wade, *Dolphin Dolphin*, Hodder & Stoughton, 1981

Dobbs, Horace, *Camera Underwater*, Focal Press, 1972

Dobbs, Horace, *Classic Dives of the World*, The Oxford Illustrated Press, 1987

Dobbs, Horace, *Dance to a Dolphin's Song*, Jonathan Cape, 1991

Dobbs, Horace, *Dilo and the Call of the Deep*, Watch Publishing, 1994

Dobbs, Horace, *Dolphin Therapy Centres: a vision for the future*, IDW, 1992

Dobbs, Horace, *Follow a Wild Dolphin*, Souvenir Press, 1990

Dobbs, Horace, *Save the Dolphins*, Souvenir Press, 1992

Dobbs, Horace, *Tale of Two Dolphins*, Jonathan Cape, 1988

Dobbs, Horace, *The Great Diving Adventure*, The Oxford Illustrated Press, 1986

Dobbs, Horace, *The Magic of Dolphins*, Lutterworth Press, 1990

Dobbs, Horace, and Sally Galotti, *Il Potere Magico di Dilo*, Parole di Cotone Edizione, 1999

Eisenberg, David, with Thomas Lee Wright, *Encounters with Qi*, Jonathan Cape, 1986

Fitzgibbon, Ronnie, *The Dingle Dolphin*, Athlone Press, 1988

Furlong, David, *The Keys to the Temple*, Piatkus Books, 1998

Gatenby, Greg (ed), *Whales – a celebration*, Little, Brown & Co., 1983

Gawain, Elizabeth, *The Dolphin's Gift*, Whatever Publishing, 1981

Goldman, Jonathan, *Healing Sounds*, Element, 1992

Hanf-Enos, Eve, and Brigitte Hanf, *I am a Hypothesis*, private publication, 1989

Hope, Murray, *The Ancient Wisdom of Atlantis*, Thorsons, 1998

Idaz, Jerry, and Michael Greenberg, *Beneath Tropic Seas*, Seahawk Press, 1987

Johnson, Jessica, and Michael Odent, *We Are All Water Babies*, Dragon's World, 1994

Kaptchuk, Ted, *Chinese Medicine*, Rider, 1993

Kewin, Joe et al, *Sensations and Disability*, Rompa, 1994

Kolosimo, Peter, *Not of This World*, Sphere Books, 1975

Layne, Libby, *The Sound of the Dolphin's Psalm*, Warwick House, 1997

Lilly, John, *Man and Dolphin*, Gollancz, 1962

Lilly, John, *The Mind of the Dolphin*, Doubleday, 1967

McCarthy, Sue, *Heaven on Earth*, The Bradbury House of Words, 1996

McIntyre, Joan, et al, *Mind in the Waters*, Scriber's, 1974

Milanovich, Norma J, and Jean Meltesen, *Sacred Journey to Atlantis*, Athena Publishing, 1994

Miller, Lana, *Call of the Dolphins*, Rainbow Bridge Publishing, 1989

Morgan, Elaine, *The Aquatic Ape*, Stein and Day, 1982

O'Sullivan, Maurice, *Twenty Years a-Growing*, OUP, 1953

Ocean, Joan, *Dolphin Connection*, Dolphin Connection, 1989

Odent, Michael, *Water and Sexuality*, Arkana, 1990

Ouwehand, Cornelius, *Hateruma: Socio-religious aspects of a south Ryukyuan island culture*, Lieden E.J. Brill, 1985

Rocha, Adriana, and Kristi Jorde, *A Child of Eternity*, Piatkus Books, 1996

Ryrie, Charlie, *The Healing Energies of Water*, Gaia Books, 1998

Sagan, Carl, *The Cosmic Connection*, Coronet, 1975

Sagan, Carl, *The Dragons of Eden*, Ballantine Books, 1978

Schul, Bill, *The Psychic Power of Animals*, Coronet, 1978

Seki, Hideo, *The Science of Higher Dimensions*, Sawayaka Publishing, 1984

Seth, Vikram, *Arion and the Dolphin*, Orion Children's Books, 1994

Shaw, Steven, *The Art of Swimming*, Ashgrove Press, 1996

St. John, Patricia, *Beyond Words*, Stillpoint Publishing, 1994

Stenuit, Robert, *The Dolphin: cousin to man*, JM. Dent and Sons, 1969

Tenzin-Dolma, Lisa, *Swimming with Dolphins*, Quantum, 1997

Tomatis, Alfred, *The Ear and Language*, Moulin Publishing, 1993

van Lippe-Biesterfield, Irene, *Dialogue with Nature*, Findhorn Press, 1998

Williams, Heathcote, *Falling for a Dolphin*, Jonathan Cape, 1990

Williams, Heathcote, *Whale Nation*, Jonathan Cape, 1988

Wiltshire, Stephen, *Cities*, JM. Dent and Sons, 1974

Wyllie, Timothy, *Dolphins, Telepathy and Underwater Birthing*, Bear & Col, 1993

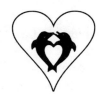

International Dolphin Watch

When I set up International Dolphin Watch (IDW) in 1978, its main function was the scientific study and conservation of dolphins. It is still staffed by part-time volunteers but its remit has broadened considerably since then. The latest information is on the website: www.idw.org.

IDW is researching dolphin healing and ways in which the benefits of swimming with dolphins can be re-created artificially – to reduce the impact on wild populations and make the experience available to severely handicapped children. IDW publishes reports and its own journal *Dolphin* which is sent free to all members. All research is non-intrusive and no studies are conducted with captive dolphins.

The Dolphin Survey Project was established at Cambridge University under Professor Sir Richard Harrison to monitor dolphin populations world-wide. IDW facilitates data input from a wide variety of professional and amateur dolphin watchers around the world. *Dolphinicity*, a research sailing boat, is monitoring cetacean populations in the North Sea and introducing people to observational and recording procedures. IDW has friendly links with organisations such as British Divers' Marine Life Rescue (BDMLR) with whom it collaborates in the rescue and treatment of stranded or injured marine mammals. IDW produces a guide on where it is possible to watch and swim with dolphins and also distributes sheets with guidelines on how to behave in the presence of dolphins. IDW actively lobbies governments world-wide – pressing for laws to be upheld where they are infringed and arguing for changes in legislation that will help protect the marine environment.

IDW publishes details of opportunities for volunteers and is actively involved in education. Its members give presentations in schools in several countries. Links are being formed with indigenous peoples, such as the Australian Aborigines, to find ways of applying their ancient wisdom and understanding of the natural world to help solve present ecological problems.

Those joining the Adopt and Watch Scheme receive an information booklet which includes details of where they *may* see their adopted dolphin free in the open sea. The IDW mail-order shop stocks a wide range of books and dolphin goodies including the *Dolphin Dreamtime* tape and CD, and *The Dolphin's Touch*, *Ride a Wild Dolphin* and *Oceania* videos.

IDW is independent and is financed by donations, bequests and subscriptions from members who become part of a friendly family of dolphin lovers. Members receive newsletters on the work of IDW which includes details of how they can become personally involved if they wish. The joining fee more or less covers the cost of printing and sending out the literature.

For further information please contact:

The Secretary
International Dolphin Watch
10 Melton Road
North Ferriby
East Yorkshire
HU14 3ET
UK

Tel: 01482 645789
Fax: 01482 634914
email: IDW@talk21.com
website: www.idw.org

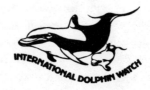

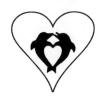

Index

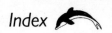

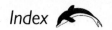

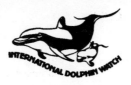

YOU CAN HELP DOLPHINS!

IDW NEEDS MEMBERS

 JOIN NOW

When you join you will receive a lovely package containing posters, copies of our magazine *Dolphin* and other exciting items.

MEMBERSHIP OF IDW
MAKES A WONDERFUL GIFT

Only £15 in the UK or £25 overseas (Annual Renewals £10 & £15)

One of the major benefits of joining IDW is that you become part of a global network. Whenever possible IDW gives out names and addresses so that you can make direct contact with those involved in the topics that interest you most.

If you are already a member please encourage a friend to join!

Enquiries, tel: 01482 645789

Name: .... Address: .... Tel:	Send your joining fee - £15 UK - £25 overseas (UK cheques or International Money Orders. Sorry no overseas cheques) to: **Membership Secretary** **International Dolphin Watch** **10 Melton Road** **North Ferriby** **East Yorkshire HU14 3ET,** **UK, and e-mail at** **idw@talk21.com**

Credit card membership accepted by fax: 01482 634914

Type: .... Name: ....

Number: ☐☐☐☐ ☐☐☐☐ ☐☐☐☐ ☐☐☐☐

Expiry Date: ☐☐ ☐☐

PIATKUS BOOKS

If you have enjoyed reading this book, you may be interested in other titles published by Piatkus. These include:

The Afterlife: An investigation into the mysteries of life after death Jenny Randles and Peter Hough

Ambika's Guide To Healing And Wholeness: The energetic path to the chakras and colour Ambika Wauters

Art Of Sexual Magic, The: How to use sexual energy to transform your life Margot Anand

As I See It: A psychic's guide to developing your healing and sensing abilities Betty F. Balcombe

Ask Your Angels: A practical guide to working with angels to enrich your life Alma Daniel, Timothy Wyllie and Andrew Ramer

At Peace In The Light: A man who died twice reveals amazing insights into life, death and its mysteries Dannion Brinkley with Paul Perry

Barefoot Doctor's Handbook For Heroes: A spiritual guide to fame and fortune Barefoot Doctor

Barefoot Doctor's Handbook For The Urban Warrior: A spiritual survival guide Barefoot Doctor

Beyond Belief: How to develop mystical consciousness and discover the God within Peter Spink

Book Of Shadows: A modern Witch reveals the wisdom of Witchcraft and the power of the Goddess Phyllis Currott

Light Up Your Life: And discover your true purpose and potential Diana Cooper

Living Magically: A new vision of reality Gill Edwards

Many Lives, Many Masters: The true story of a prominent psychiatrist, his young patient and the past-life therapy that changed both of their lives Dr Brian L. Weiss

Mary's Message To The World Annie Kirkwood

Meditation For Every Day: Includes over 100 inspiring meditations for busy people Bill Anderton

Message Of Love, A: A channelled guide to our future Ruth White

Messenger, The: The journey of a spiritual teacher Geoff Boltwood

Mindfulness Meditation For Everyday Life Jon Kabat-Zinn

Miracles: A collection of true stories which prove that miracles do happen Cassandra Eason

Nostradamus: The next 50 years Peter Lemesurier

Nostradamus: The final reckoning Peter Lemesurier

One Last Time: A psychic medium speaks to those we have loved and lost John Edward

Only Love Is Real: A story of soulmates reunited Dr Brian L. Weiss

Paranormal Source Book, The: The comprehensive guide to strange phenomena worldwide Jenny Randles

Parting Visions: An exploration of predeath psychic and spiritual experiences Dr Melvin Morse with Paul Perry

Past Lives, Present Dreams: How to use reincarnation for personal growth Denise Linn

Past Lives, Future Lives Jenny Cockell

Peter Underwood's Guide To Ghosts And Haunted Places Peter Underwood

Pocketful Of Dreams: The mysterious world of dreams revealed Denise Linn

Secret Language Of Dreams, The: A visual key to dreams and their meanings David Fontana

Secret Language Of Symbols, The: A visual key to symbols and their meanings David Fontana

Secret World Of Your Dreams, The Derek and Julia Parker

Serpent And The Circle, The: A practical guide to shamanism Namua Rahesha

Stepping Into The Magic: A new approach to everyday life Gill Edwards

Supernatural Britain: A guide to Britain's most haunted locations Peter Hough

Talking To Heaven: A medium's message of life after death James Van Praagh

Tarot Made Easy Nancy Garen

Teach Yourself To Meditate: Over 20 simple exercises for peace, health and clarity of mind Eric Harrison

Thoughts That Harm, Thoughts That Heal: Overcoming common ailments through the power of your mind Keith Mason

Three Minute Meditator, The: 30 simple ways to relax and unwind David Harp with Nina Feldman

Time For Healing, A: The journey to wholeness Eddie and Debbie Shapiro

Time For Transformation, A: How to awaken to your soul's purpose and claim your power Diana Cooper

Toward A Meaningful Life: The wisdom of the Rebbe Menachem Mendel Schneerson Simon Jacobson (ed.)

Transformed By The Light: The powerful effect of near-death experiences on people's lives Dr Melvin Morse with Paul Perry

Transform Your Life: A step-by-step programme for change Diana Cooper

Vibrational Medicine For The 21st Century: A complete guide to energy healing and spiritual transformation Richard Gerber MD

Visualisation: An introductory guide Helen Graham

Way Of Harmony, The: How to find true abundance in your life Jim Dreaver

Working With Guides And Angels Ruth White

Working With Your Chakras Ruth White

World Mythology: The illustrated guide Dr Roy Willis

Yesterday's Children: The extraordinary search for my past-life family Jenny Cockell

Yin And Yang: Understanding the Chinese philosophy of opposites and how to apply it to your everyday life Martin Palmer

Your Body Speaks Your Mind: Understand how your thoughts and emotions affect your health Debbie Shapiro

Your Healing Power: A comprehensive guide to channelling your healing abilities Jack Angelo

For a free brochure with our complete list of titles, please write to:

Piatkus Books
5 Windmill Street
London W1P 1HF
Tel: 020 7631 0710
Email: *info@piatkus.co.uk*
Website: *www.piatkus.co.uk*

PIATKUS